The
Palliative
Response

F. Amos Bailey, M.D.

Published by Menasha Ridge Press
Printed in the United States of America
Second edition, Second Printing

ISBN 0-89732-968-6

Cataloging-in-Publication Data available from the Library of Congress

Text design by Jennie Zehmer
Cover design by Lori Pandy and Travis Bryant

Disclaimer

The information in this book is intended as a guideline. The author and the publisher do not accept any legal responsibility or liability for any errors in the text or misuse or misapplication of material in the book. All health-care providers should exercise independent clinical judgment and consult the official prescribing information before the use of any product.

Table of Contents

Acknowledgments

The Palliative Response represents the encouragement and support of many individuals who deserve recognition and who, I hope, will be honored by this work. I owe foremost gratitude to the patients who have been my primary teachers over the last 15 years. In the classrooms of their homes and hospital rooms, they have taught me much! It is a great privilege to be invited into a home; it is really being invited into a life. For allowing me that privilege, I thank Ms. M., my first hospice patient about whom I write in the Preface, and the over 2000 people on whom I since have made house calls. Palliative-care inpatients, first at the Balm of Gilead Center at Cooper Green Hospital and now at the Safe Harbor Project at the Birmingham Veterans Administration Medical Center, have all been wonderful educators. It is my honor to pass on their many lessons.

Dr. William Dismukes, Residency Director at UAB Health Systems, planted the seed for this book in 1999 when he asked that all Balm of Gilead patients be assigned to residents, and invited me to devote the final 10–15 minutes of each morning report to palliative care. Suddenly, I had a forum in which to talk about palliative care, and these talks gradually became *The Palliative Response*. My appreciation goes to the residents and medical students assigned to the Cooper Green Hospital Medical Service, who have listened and responded to these talks for the last four years.

My deep appreciation goes to Cooper Green Hospital and its former CEO Dr. Max Michel, who believed that we could create the Balm of Gilead Center as a site of excellence for End-of-Life care and training, and to all my colleagues at the Balm of Gilead and the Birmingham Area Hospice. Together we believed in a vision, and together we nurtured the vision into excellent care in the hospital and hospice of a public health system. Palliative Specialist/Nurse Practitioner Edwina Taylor, RN, CRNP; Project Director James Bolden, MPA, MT (ASCP); Charge Nurse Barbara Sunday, RN; and Community Coordinator Carol Padgett, PhD were instrumental in helping shape the Balm of Gilead into a community of caring at the End of Life.

Dr. Ira Byock and the Robert Wood Johnson Foundation, who selected Cooper Green Hospital and the Balm of Gilead as a demonstration project for Promoting Excellence in End-of-Life care, have offered unwavering support. Their emphasis on dissemination has inspired me to find ways to share the things we have learned and are continuing to learn about palliative care. Dr. Byock's focus on the potential at Life's End for growth in both patients and their caregivers sustains my motivation and guides my interactions.

Carol Padgett has helped organize my material while lending her insights as a keen observer of palliative patients, the human condition, and my interactions with patients, families, staff, and students.

My wife Marci and my children Mandy, Patrick, and Lydia faithfully sent me to my desk to write and faithfully appeared with technical support when the computer went on the fritz. My deepest gratitude, however, is reserved for their moral support, which has made all the difference.

— Dr. F. Amos Bailey,
Birmingham, September 2003

About the Author

In his preface to *The Palliative Response* the author poses the apparent paradox of growth at the end of life. To track the career of F. Amos Bailey is to examine a paradigm of professional growth. This career has taken him from his training as a medical oncologist to a practice in a small Appalachian community to an inner-city public hospital (where he founded the Balm of Gilead, an inpatient hospice facility) to a hospital for veterans. Through those transitions F. Amos Bailey has "morphed" from a simple practitioner of the healing arts into an icon for a new model of medicine's primary mission, the relief of human suffering.

Along the way, Dr. Bailey has become a teacher. He is, however, quite unlike the typical clinical educators who populate the corridors of modern teaching hospitals. Many of them are drawn to their work by a love of the academic environment and a fascination with the process of learning. F. Amos Bailey has been compelled to teach by the desire to advance the mission of palliative care and the need to touch more patients whose suffering needs his balm.

In an era when translation research is a key phrase for priority funding, F. Amos Bailey is perhaps the ultimate "translationalist." He has taken a body of clinically relevant knowledge from multiple domains and demonstrated how to apply it at the bedside in new way. Through this book he shows us how we can be better doctors.

F. Amos Bailey lives and grows in Birmingham with his wife Marci, and their children Mandy, Patrick, and Lydia. He currently practices his art at the VA Medical Center, where he directs the Safe Harbor Palliative Care Project.

— Dr. John I. Kennedy, Jr.
Associate Chief of Staff for Primary Care, Birmingham, VAMC
Professor of Medicine, Division of Pulmonary and Critical Care Medicine, University of Alabama, Birmingham

Preface

Growing Pains

*Maslow, Erickson, and Piaget each told us
that human development is a lifelong process.
I think it simply turns out that they were right.*

—Ira Byock, M.D.

Growth at the Life's End? Such an idea initially might sound like an oxymoron. Life's End is, after all, a euphemism for Death. What could growth and death have to do with each other? I find part of the answer to that question in the concept of "growing pains." Some children experience pain in their bones at times in their lives when the growth is rapid, sudden and unexpected. When nothing else can explain the pain, we shrug and diagnose "growing pains."

This palliative-care manual is the fruit of "growing pains." In 1989, I moved to Beckley, West Virginia. I had completed training in Medical Oncology and had chosen to practice in a little Appalachian town to test my mettle and ability. Nothing in ten years of training, including a Medical Oncology Fellowship, had prepared me for the immediate turn that my professional life took toward providing care where there can be no cure. A patient, guided by a women's magazine and the wisdom of personal experience, taught me more about caring for the dying than I had learned from mentors guided by medical texts and the tenets of professional practice. Only when I happened upon the *Oxford Textbook of Palliative Medicine* did I recognize that "the suffering paradigm" had been the template over our discussions.

During my first month of private practice in West Virginia, a nurse and social worker asked me to serve as Medical Director for the hospice they hoped to start, assuring me that my duties would include only "signing some papers and writing a few prescriptions for pain medicine." During my second month, I was summoned to the home of Ms. M., who a year earlier had noticed numbness in her right hand. The CT scan had shown a tumor and the biopsy had confirmed its malignancy. Although radiation had held things in check for a few months, the numbness recurred and the repeat scan only confirmed what everyone knew was the recurrence of her cancer and the beginning of the end. Ms. M. read about hospice in "a women's magazine," requested a referral, and identified me as her "new doctor." Following the article's description of hospice care, which she was sure included house calls, Ms. M. was now demanding that her new doctor see her at her home.

With great trepidation, I made my way to her residence. What could I do for her? How could I help her in her own home? In ten years of training, I had received no formal instruction in caring for the dying. I had never referred a patient to hospice and had never heard the words "palliative care." On more than one occasion, I had witnessed patients dying while chemotherapy was being infused into their veins.

Entering Ms. M.'s home, I found a moon-faced bald woman propped in her chair and gazing into her backyard. Ms. M. was gracious and introduced me to her family. I dealt with a few minor adjustments in her medicines. And then she asked me what might happen. She discussed concerns about her children and about unfinished tasks, her interest in meditation and her childhood Catholic faith. She spoke of sadness and fears and, as we ended, told me how much I had helped and asked me to return soon. I visited Ms. M. for the next few months, until she died one cold fall night in her own home surrounded by her family.

I now understand my experience with Ms. M. as one of pain and growth for all who were involved. For me it was an epiphany. Over the next few years, amazed at how much better my dying patients fared at home than in the hospital, I strove to arrange for them to be discharged so that their suffering could be eased; and my clinical interventions in the hospital and clinics became tempered with home-style comfort care. All the while, I remained frustrated at the host of barriers that prevented greater application during hospital care of lessons learned from home care.

I have worked with many teachers since Ms. M. They have included my patients and colleagues in West Virginia, later at the Balm of Gilead Project at Cooper Green Hospital, and now at the Birmingham Veterans Administration Medical Center. This palliative-care manual is a distillation of some of the lessons I am learning.

Life's End can be a time of growth for each of us. Persons who are facing a life-threatening or terminal illness have been "dying" since the day they were born. Now, however, that reality thrusts its way to center stage and demands attention. The dying process can be a time of personal growth for these persons, their families and all with whom they come in contact. Dying persons and their communities grow as they accommodate the changes that are inevitable as death approaches. Palliative care can help each of us to experience personal growth in the light of Life's End. No one can make anyone grow. However, excellent end-of-life care—care that alleviates some of the physical, emotional, social, and spiritual suffering of Life's End—can allow patients, families, and their community of caring to grow and even blossom.

About This Book

As Medical Director of the Balm of Gilead Palliative Care Unit at Cooper Green Hospital, I supervised the General Internal Medicine residents who followed all patients admitted to the unit. The need for basic education in palliative care became clear shortly after the initiation of "palliative work rounds" during the final 15 minutes of the residents' Daily Morning Report. The chapters in this manual are the fruits of this opportunity to introduce new physicians to key dimensions of palliative care.

The manual's topics, designed for presentations of 12–15 minutes, cover management of physical symptoms and emotional, spiritual, and social issues common in end-of-life care. The manual offers guidance for specific palliative roles, such as sharing bad news, conducting a family conference, and making a death pronouncement. Chapters on specific diseases review common symptoms, end-of-life manifestations, and prognostic signs that might prompt referral to palliative care and hospice.

Each chapter opens with annotated **Key Points** from the 12–15 minute discussion and continues with a more detailed **Handout.** Each chapter concludes with **Selected Readings** that direct the student to references for further study on the chapter's topic.

The manual is appropriate as a basic classroom text for students and as a tutorial guide for residents and fellows in Palliative Medicine rotations. Its form facilitates selecting relevant sections for integration into classroom teaching or for review by rounding groups or consulting residents.

Five **Provider Pocket Cards** accompany the manual:

Consider Palliative Medicine outlines the conditions and goals warranting palliative-care consultation.

Analgesic Dosing is an aid for pain management.

Sharing Bad News/Family Conference offers a procedure for speaking with patients and families about realities and decisions associated with Life's End.

Last Hours of Life suggests orders appropriate for patient comfort and family support.

Guidelines for Death Pronouncement leads the physician through the interpersonal and technical aspects of pronouncement, documentation, and follow-up family contacts.

My goal in developing *The Palliative Response* has been to offer a concise and accessible package suitable for palliative-care instruction and review in a variety of settings. My larger hope is that this effort will help bolster the competence, confidence, and commitment of medical providers to integrate *The Palliative Response* into daily clinical practice. I would appreciate feedback and constructive criticism from colleagues so that future revisions will reflect the ongoing refinement of palliative principles and practice.

Introduction to Palliative Care

Introduction to Palliative Care

Key Points

1. Palliative Care is a holistic response to suffering in the physical, emotional, social, and spiritual domains.

2. It is appropriate to integrate aggressive palliative management of symptoms into the care of patients receiving disease-modifying therapy.

3. Ninety percent of Americans would prefer to receive care at Life's End in their homes rather than in hospitals or nursing homes.

4. Instead, 50% of persons dying in the United States die in hospitals, 25% in nursing homes, 15% in personal homes, and 10% suddenly outside the hospital.

5. Home Hospice is a Medicare-defined benefit program that provides palliative care for some patients at home. Only 15–20% of dying persons are referred to hospice, and usually for less than the last month of life.

Introduction to Palliative Care

Suffering Paradigm

Social

Physical **Suffering** Emotional

Spiritual

End of Life in America:
What Do People Want?

Gallup Poll Results:
Nine out of 10 people would prefer to die at home if terminally ill with six months or less to live

70% would seek hospice care
62% would seek curative care

End of Life in America:
Where/How Do We Die?

- 15% die at home
- 10% die unexpectedly
- 25% die in nursing homes
- 50% die in hospitals

Why People Die
Causes of Death

- Heart Disease
- Cancer
- Stroke

Account for 67% of the deaths in people 65 years of age and older

---

Palliative Care
What Is It?

- Prevention and relief of symptoms
- Attention to emotional and spiritual needs
- Care for the patient and family as a unit
- Sensitive communication, goal setting and advance planning
- Interdisciplinary care
- Services appropriate to the various settings in which people die

Hospice
What Is It?

- A program to provide palliative care when life expectancy is six months or less
- Covered by Medicare and Medicaid
- Covered by private insurance plans with enhanced home-care benefits

Physical Suffering:
The Palliative Response

- Pain and multiple non-pain symptoms

  Treat pain; it is frequently undertreated.

  Assess/treat other sources of physical distress.
- Symptom prevention

  Foster compliance with treatment.
- Advance planning

  Collaborate with patient and caregivers.

  Anticipate and plan for likely events.

Emotional Suffering:
The Palliative Response

- Depression
- Anxiety
- Delirium
- Loneliness

Social Suffering:
The Palliative Response

- Limited income
- Lack of insurance

  Insurance often does not cover prescription medicines and home health services.
- Inadequate housing
- Social isolation
- Caregiver fatigue

Spiritual Suffering:
The Palliative Response

- Loss of hope
- Inability to sustain relations with faith community
- Search for meaning

The Palliative Response

Every physician
needs to know
the palliative response

Introduction to Palliative Care

Selected Readings

Palliative Care Overview

Billings, J. A. "Palliative care: definitions and controversy." In *Principles & Practice of Supportive Oncology,* edited by A. M. Berger, R. K. Portenoy, D. E. Weissman. New York: Lipincott Williams & Wilkins Healthcare, 1998.

Cassell, E. J. "Diagnosing Suffering: A Perspective." *Annals of Internal Medicine* 131 (1999): 531–534.

Cassel, E. J. "The nature of suffering and the goals of medicine." *The New England Journal of Medicine* 306 (1982): 639–645.

History of Palliative Care

Saunders, C: "Into the Valley of the Shadow of Death: A Personal Therapeutic Journey." *British Medical Journal* 313 (1996): 1599–1601.

SUPPORT Principal Investigators: A controlled Trial to Improve Care for Seriously Ill Hospitalized Patients: The Study to Understand Prognoses and Preferences for Outcomes and Risks of Treatments (SUPPORT). *The Journal of American Medical Association* 274 (1995): 1591–1598.

Predominance of the Curative Model

Fox, E. "Predominance of the Curative Model of Medical Care: A Residual Problem." *The Journal of American Medical Association* 278 (1997): 761–763.

Morrison, R. S., D. E. Meier, and D. E. Cassel. "When Too Much Is Too Little." *The New England Journal of Medicine* 335 (1996): 1755–1759.

In Search of a Good Death

Byock, I. R. "Nature of Suffering and the Nature of Opportunity at the End of Life." *Clinics in Geriatric Medicine* 12 (1996): 237–253.

Steinhauser, K. E., E. C. Clipp, M. McNeilly, N. A. Christakis, L. M. McIntyre, and J. A. Tulsky: "In Search of a Good Death: Observations of Patients, Families, and Providers." *Annals of Internal Medicine* 132 (2000): 825–832.

Physical Suffering: The Palliative Response

1.1 Anorexia

Key Points

1. Anorexia is a manifestation of the underlying disease.

     Anorexia is not the cause of the patient's terminal condition.
   However, most families and physicians express this erroneous belief
   in statements such as, "If only he would eat, he would get better!"

2. Family and friends are often more concerned than the patient
   about anorexia.

     Providers can help family and friends find alternative ways to
   express their love and concern, so that eating does not become an
   area of conflict.

3. Anorexia may have multiple causes related to poor symptom
   control.

     The provider can look for reversible causes of anorexia, such as
   poorly controlled pain and other physical symptoms, and can seek
   the help of dietary professionals in selecting palatable foods. A
   "cardiac prudent diet" is probably no longer necessary.

4. Anorexia may respond to an appetite stimulant like dexamethasone.

     Dexamethasone is a preferred appetite stimulant. It is effective,
   inexpensive, and may have additional benefits such as serving as an
   adjunct for pain control, lifting the patient's mood, and addressing
   asthenia. Megestrol is expensive ($300–$500/month), not very
   effective, and results in no identifiable improvement in quality
   of life.

5. Anorexia, when severe, often results in the use of IVF, TPN, or tube
   feedings.

     These treatments may be very appropriate to bridge and support
   someone until normal eating can resume. For most people at the
   Life's End, these treatments can cause:

     1) iatrogenic harm because of infections, fluid overload, and
   aspiration pneumonia;

     2) pain and discomfort from the placement and maintenance of
   IV and tubes;

     3) increased use of restraints to protect IV lines and feeding
   tubes.

Anorexia

The Palliative Response

Anorexia Is a Symptom

Anorexia is a common symptom at Life's End.

Decreased intake is nearly universal in the last few weeks to days of life.

The Role of the Physician

- Look for reversible causes
- Consider the use of appetite stimulants
- Provide accurate and helpful information
- Help family members identify alternative methods of expressing love
- Ensure that any IV or tube feedings are safe, effective, and consistent with Goals of Care

Dietary Management

- Involve the patient in menu planning
- Offer small portions of patient's favorite foods
- Offer easy-to-swallow foods
- Try sweets
- Avoid foods with strong smells, flavor, or spices, unless patient requests

Responding to Family Concerns

- Family members and caregivers are more concerned about lack of appetite and may harass the patient about decreased intake
- Anticipate family concerns and initiate family discussion about decreased appetite
- Be prepared to discuss and review this symptom every time you meet with family
- Demonstrate willingness to look for reversible causes and to use appetite stimulants

Educating Patient and Family

about progression of the underlying illness and its effect on appetite

- Anorexia is a symptom of the disease
- The patient is not starving
- Forced feeding often causes discomfort
- Artificial feeding usually does not prolong life and may shorten it
- Patients are usually not uncomfortable from decreased intake and can live for long periods on little food

Reversible Causes of Anorexia
Differential Considerations

- Poorly controlled pain and non-pain symptoms
- Nausea and vomiting
- GI dysmotility (gastroparesis)
- Oral infections such as thrush or herpes simplex
- Xerostomia (dry mouth)

Reversible Causes of Anorexia
Differential Considerations

- Constipation and urinary retention
- Medications such as iron supplements
- Chemotherapy and radiation
- Depression and anxiety
- Gastritis and Peptic Ulcer Disease

Consider an Appetite Stimulant
Alcohol

- Wine, sherry, and beer have significant calories and are well-known appetite stimulants
- Consider using if consistent with culture and heritage and if no history of past alcohol abuse
- Many people who had used alcohol routinely before they became ill have the impression that they must now not drink alcohol at all

Consider an Appetite Stimulant
Cyproheptadine (Periactin)

- This antihistamine has the side effect of weight gain
- Has been used to treat anorexia nervosa
- Not highly effective and may be more placebo effect than active drug
- Is not likely to be helpful at Life's End

Consider an Appetite Stimulant
Megestrol (Megase)

- Approved for the treatment of AIDS wasting
- Dose for wasting is megestrol suspension 800mg QD
- Expensive—approximately $350/month
- Major side effects are Pulmonary embolism nausea and vomiting

Consider an Appetite Stimulant
Megestrol (Megase)

- In patients with cancer, the use of megestrol was not associated with any documented improvement in QOL or survival
- Usually not recommend for anorexia at EOL

Consider an Appetite Stimulant
Dexamethasone (Decadron)

- Dose of 2–4mg at breakfast and lunch
- Can tell within a few days to a week if effective
- Inexpensive
- May also have beneficial effects on pain, asthenia, and mood
- Causes less fluid retention than other corticosteroids

Consider an Appetite Stimulant
Dexamethasone (Decadron)

- Use caution with history of diabetes mellitus
- Usually not concerned in the EOL setting about long-term complications of steroids
- May be a good choice in COPD patients who have become steroid dependent

Consider an Appetite Stimulant
Dronabinol (Marinol)

- Usually used in young patients with past experience with marijuana
- Expensive—up to $500/month
- Requires DEA Schedule III
- Usually used in HIV or as part of treatment protocol with chemotherapy

Artificial Nutrition at Life's End
Tube Feeding

- Tube feeding and forced feeding in terminally ill patients have not been shown to prolong life
- Nasogastric and gastrostomy tube feedings are associated with:
  Aspiration pneumonia
  Self-extubation and thus use of restraints
  Nausea and diarrhea
  Rattling and increased respiratory secretions

Artificial Nutrition at Life's End
Total Parenteral Nutrition (TPN)

Meta-analysis of 12 randomized trials in cancer patients (1980s)
- Decreased survival
- Decreased response to chemotherapy
- Increased rate of infections

*Is anorexia ever
a protective mechanism?*

Artificial Nutrition at Life's End
Consider Potential Burdens

Tube feeding and IV hydration often increase secretions, ascites, and effusions, which require additional treatments.

*Always ask:
"Are these kinds of treatments in line with the Goals of Care?"*

Selected Readings

Myths, Theories, and Decision-Making

Cross, K. L. "If He Would Just Eat, I Know He Would Get Stronger." *Quarterly Newsletter of the American Academy of Hospice and Palliative Medicine* 1 (2001): 12–14.

Medical Management

Bruera, E. "ABC of Palliative Care: Anorexia, Cachexia, and Nutrition." *British Medical Journal* 315 (1997): 1219–1222.

Jatoi, A. and C. L. Loprinzi. "Current Management of Cancer-Associated Anorexia and Weight Loss." *Oncology* 15 (2001): 497–509.

Jatoi, A., H. E.Windschitl, C. L. Loprinzi, J. A. Sloan, S. R. Dakhil, J. A. Mailliard, R. Pundaleeka, C. G. Kardinal, T. R. Fitch, J. E. Krook, P. J. Novotny, and B. Christensen. "Dronobinal versus Megestrol Acetate versus Combination Therapy for Cancer-Associated Anorexia: A North Central Cancer Treatment Group Study." *Journal of Clinical Oncology* 20 (2002): 567–573.

1.2 Asthenia (Fatigue)

Key Points

1. The subjective and multidimensional symptoms of Asthenia cause ongoing distress in more than 90% of people at Life's End.

   Asthenia is prevalent with chemotherapy or radiation and persistent or progressive cancers, universal with the biologic response modifiers, and common with many other illnesses with end organ failure.

2. Assess fatigue by asking patient about its presence, severity, interference with activities, level of concern, and impact on Quality of Life.

   Cognitive complaints include short-term memory loss and diminished concentration and attention. Emotional complaints include marked reactivity to feeling fatigued and decreased motivation and interest in usual activities. Practical complaints include difficulty completing tasks, struggle to overcome inactivity, and post-exertional malaise lasting several hours.

3. The pathophysiology of fatigue requires differential diagnosis that evaluates also for progressive cancer, intercurrent systemic disease, and other causal factors.

   Such factors include sleep disorders, deconditioning and immobility, central-acting drugs, chronic pain or other poorly controlled symptoms, depression and anxiety.

4. Manage fatigue according to stage of underlying illness, effects of treatment, changing Goals of Care, and life expectancy.

   Stop nonessential medications. Try to avoid invasive enteral and parenteral routes when hydrating or feeding. Look for easily correctable metabolic disorders. Hydration and food supplements may help.

5. Dexamethasone is the preferred steroid at Life's End and may be helpful for fatigue in the late stages of illness.

   Its effect may last 2–3 months, and it has less mineral-corticoid effect. Dexamethasone 4mg po ~ Prednisone 15mg po.

6. Counsel fatigued patient to set realistic goals, conserve energy for most important activities, exercise, and practice good sleep hygiene.

Asthenia (Fatigue)

The Palliative Response

Impact

- Reported by > 90% of persons at Life's End
- Often most distressing symptom, even compared to pain or anorexia
- Limits activity
- Increases dependency
- Diminishes sense of control, and self-determination

Prevalence

- Universal with biologic response modifiers
- > 96% with chemotherapy or radiation
- > 90% with persistent or progressive cancers
- Common with many other illnesses with end organ failure

  (Congestive Heart Failure, Chronic Pulmonary Disease, Chronic Renal Failure, General Debility)

Characteristics

- Subjective
  Severity
  Distress
  Time Line
- Multidimensional
  Weakness and or lack of energy
  Sleepiness
  Difficulty concentrating

Patient Experience
Physical Symptoms

- Generalized weakness
- Limb heaviness
- Sleep disturbances
  Insomnia
  Hypersomnia
  Unrefreshing/nonrestorative sleep

Patient Experience
Cognitive Symptoms

- Short-term memory loss
- Diminished concentration
- Diminished attention

Patient Experience
Emotional Symptoms

- Marked emotional reactivity to fatigue
- Decreased motivation/interest in usual activities

Patient Experience
Practical

- Difficulty completing daily tasks
- Struggle to overcome inactivity
- Post-exertional malaise lasting several hours

Differential Diagnosis
Potential Mechanisms of Asthenia Associated with Cancer

- Progressive disease
- Cytokines
- Decreased metabolic substrates
- Change in energy metabolism
- Treatments
  Chemotherapy, radiation, surgery, and biologics
  Effects are cumulative and can last for months

Differential Diagnosis
Intercurrent Systemic Disease

- Anemia
- Infections
- Malnutrition
- Dehydration and electrolyte imbalance

Differential Diagnoses

- Sleep disorders
- Deconditioning and immobility
- Central-acting drugs
- Chronic pain/other poorly controlled symptoms
- Depression
- Anxiety

Assessment

- Do you have fatigue?
- How severe is your fatigue? (Use analog scale)
- Does fatigue interfere with activities?
- Are you worried about the fatigue?
- Does fatigue impact your Quality of Life? How?

Goals of Care

- Fatigue usually remains a concern throughout stages of illness at Life's End (although may respond in part to treatment)
- Modify Goals of Care by stage of illness
  Prolongation of life or cure of disease
  Improving function
  Comfort and supportive care

Effect on Fatigue
Disease-Modifying Therapies

- Some therapies may worsen fatigue
  Chemotherapy or radiation for cancer

- Others may improve fatigue
  Dialysis for renal failure
  ACE for congestive heart failure
  Oxygen for hypoxia
  Opioids for pain management

Anemia in Cancer Patients
Benefits of Erythropoetin (EPO)

Placebo Controlled Trial
Subjects randomized to EPO
Hemoglobin 8–10g/dl

- Increased hemoglobin
- Decreased use of transfusion
- Increased Quality of Life
- Effects independent of tumor response

Anemia in Cancer Patients
Burdens of EPO

- Requires injections
  (EPO 10,000 units subcutaneous 3 times a week)
- Expensive and insurance may not cover $400–$500/month
- Variable effectiveness
  Takes weeks to be effective
  May require higher doses for effect
  Not always effective

Management of Fatigue

- Stop all nonessential medications
- Look for easily correctable metabolic disorders (e.g., decreased potassium or magnesium levels)
- Hydration and food supplements may be helpful (usually try to avoid invasive enteral and parenteral routes)

Management of Fatigue
Associated with Depression

- Symptoms of major depression
  Depressed mood
  Anxiety
  Irritability
- Treatment (choice depends on life expectancy)
  SSRI's
  Counseling
  Psycho-stimulants
  Supportive management

Management of Fatigue
Dexamethasone

- May be helpful in late stages of illness
- Effect may last for 2–3 months
- A preferred steroid in this setting
  Less mineral-corticoid effect

  Prednisone results in more edema

  Dexamethasone 4mg po ~ Prednisone 15mg po

Use of Dexamethasone

- Dosage
  Dexamethasone 4–8mg q am
  May increase to 16mg qd (equivalent to Prednisone 60mg)
  Usually no advantage to higher doses
  Avoid nighttime dosing because of insomnia
- Side effects
  Watch for side effects, although they are usually well tolerated
  Long-term complications usually not a concern

Management of Fatigue
Sleep Hygiene

- Use Trazedone (25–100mg q hs) for insomnia instead of benzodiazepine
- Avoid napping
- Avoid stimulants in the evening
- Avoid alcohol before bed
- Exercise during the day (even sitting up in chair)

Management of Fatigue
Education/Counseling

- Goal setting
  Assist patient to set realistic goals.
- Energy conservation
  Counsel saving energy for most important activities.
- Assistance with activities of daily living
  Enlist the assistance of family.
  Home Health Aide and Homemaker PT/OT evaluation for appliances and exercise

Management of Fatigue
Exercise

- Physical Therapy (PT)
  Evaluate appropriateness of PT to improve quality, and perhaps even quantity, of life for patients with better prognosis.
- Up Out of Bed
  Can significantly impact QOL for patients at Life's End
  Range of motion to maintain flexibility

Asthenia at Life's End

Fatigue, weakness, and lack of stamina cause suffering in > 90% of persons at Life's End.

Asthenia (Fatigue)

Selected Readings

Overview of the Symptom of Asthenia

Chang C.H., A. Peterman, and M. Slavin. "Fatigue in Cancer Patients Compared with Fatigue in the General United States Population." *Cancer* 94 (2002): 11.

Manzullo, E. F. and C. P. Escalante. "Research into Fatigue." (review) [47 refs]. *Hematology/Oncology Clinics of North America* 16 (2002): 619–628.

Rosseau, P. "Asthenia in Terminally Ill Cancer Patients: A brief Review." *American Journal of Hospice and Palliative Care* 14 (1997): 258–261.

Stone, P., J. Hardy, K. Broadley, A. J. Tookman, A. Kurowska, and R. A'Hern. "Fatigue in Advanced Cancer: A Prospective Controlled Cross-Sectional Study." *British Journal of Cancer* 79 (1999): 1479–86.

Evaluation and Management of Asthenia

Portenoy, R. K. and L. M. Itri. "Cancer-Related Fatigue: Guidelines for Evaluation and Management." *The Oncologist* 4 (1999): 1–10.

Scialla, A., R. Cole, T. Scialla, L. Bednarz, and J. Scheerer: "Rehabilitation for Elderly Patients with Cancer Asthenia: Making a Transition to Palliative Care." *Palliative Medicine* 14 (2000): 121–127.

1.3 Constipation

Key Points

1. Assess all patients at Life's End for constipation. Evaluate for obstipation after 48 hours without a bowel movement.

   Over half of patients at Life's End suffer from constipation. Inquire about bowel habits (frequency, consistency, and previous habits), other symptoms (nausea/vomiting, abdominal pain, distention, anorexia, and diet), and attempted interventions. Obstipation is such severe constipation and impaction that there is a functional bowel obstruction.

2. Determine the cause of constipation by rectal digital exam, abdominal exam, and neurological exam. Radiographic and laboratory studies may be helpful.

   Rectal exam: Evaluate for impaction, hemorrhoids, or other problems. Abdominal exam: Evaluate for bladder distention, hernias, and masses.

3. Asthenia (fatigue) can play a role in constipation at Life's End by disrupting the normal gastrocolic reflex and limiting activity and privacy.

   Support bowel routine. Assist patient to be up. Assist to the toilet when urge occurs. Serve hot beverages. Assure as much privacy as possible.

4. Differential diagnosis should consider medication side effects, concurrent diseases, and environmental factors.

5. Physicians should treat constipation rather than withholding opioids that may be contributory.

6. Large-bowel stimulants and interventions to support bowel routine are key to managing constipation in the palliative-care setting.

   Over 80% of palliative patients, and nearly all on opioids, require laxative therapy. Use Bisacodyl (Dulcolax) 1–4 tablets a day or Senna 2–8 tablets a day. Senna can be much more expensive—be guided by patient preference.

Constipation

The Palliative Response

Overview of Constipation

- Definition

  The infrequent passage of small hard feces

- Prevalence at Life's End

  Over half of palliative care patients report constipation as a troubling symptom

- Intervention

  >80% of patients at Life's End need laxatives

  Nearly all patients on opioids need laxatives

Assess Constipation
in All Palliative Patients

- Bowel Habits

  Frequency and consistency

  Previous bowel habits

- Other Symptoms

  Nausea/vomiting

  Abdominal pain, distention, anorexia

- Interventions

  What has been tried and what helps?

Assess for Impaction

- General Rule

  Evaluate for constipation and impaction after 48 hours with no bowel movement

- Obstipation

  Functional bowel obstruction from severe constipation and impaction

Asthenia (Fatigue)
as Contributor

- Disruption of normal gastrocolic reflex

  Gastrocolic reflex produces urge to defecate usually within an hour after breakfast and lunch

  Urge will resolve in 10–15 minutes if suppressed

  Reflex may disappear if suppressed for several days

- Limited activity

  Often cannot walk to the bathroom

- Limited privacy

  Prevents or deters use of bedside commode/bedpan

Support Bowel Routine

- Assist patient with being up
- Hot beverage if known to be helpful
- Assist patient to toilet when urge occurs
- Assure as much privacy as possible

Rectal Digital Exam

- Tumor
- Constipation
- Impaction
- Local fissures
- Hemorrhoids
- Ulcers

Abdominal Exam

- Bladder distention
- Urinary retention
- Obstruction
- Hernias
- Masses
  Tumor
  Impacted stool

Additional Evaluation

- Neurological exam
  Impending cord compression
- Consider flat plate and upright X-rays
  High impaction
  Bowel obstruction
  Gastric outlet obstruction
- Lab evaluation
  Hypercalcemia
  Hypokalemia

Differential Diagnosis
Medication Review

- Opioids
- Medications with anticholinergic effects
- Diuretics
- Iron
- Anticonvulsants and anti-hypertensives
- Vincristine and platinols
- Antacids with calcium and aluminum
- Ondanstron

Continuation of Opioids

- Treat constipation rather than withdrawing opioids
- Never stop opioids as response to constipation if patient requires opioids for relief of pain or other distressing symptoms

Differential Diagnosis
Concurrent Diseases

- Diabetes
- Hypothyroidism
- Hyperparathyroidism
- Hypokalemia and hypomagnesemia
- Hernia
- Diverticular disease
- Anal fissures and stenosis
- Hemorrhoids

Differential Diagnosis
Environmental Factors

- Decreased food intake
- Dehydration
- Weakness and inactivity
- Confusion
- Depression
- Structural barriers to bathroom or toilet

Laxative Treatments

- Softeners
  Surfactants like docusate (Colase)
- Osmotic
  Lactulose
  Sorbitol
- Bulking agents
  Metamucil (usually not appropriate at EOL)
- Saline laxative
  Magnesium citrates or Milk of Magnesia (MOM)

Large Bowel Stimulant

Constipation must be managed in the palliative-care setting

- Bisacodyl (Dulcolax) 1–4 tablets a day
- Senna 2–8 tablets a day
  Can be much more expensive than bisacodyl
  Be guided by patient preference

Algorithm for Treatment

Rectal Exam ──────┐
         │   Soft feces
   Impaction
      │
Consider oil retention
enema to soften feces

Spontaneous defecation of Impaction	Manual Disimpaction Consider sedation with Lorazepam
Soft feces	Soft feces

Algorithm for Treatment

Soft feces
│
Base choice of treatment on:

- Patient preference
- Urgency for bowel movement

Oral Biscodyl or Magnesium Citrate	Fleets Enema or Biscodyl Suppository
Rectal vault empty	Rectal vault empty

Algorithm for Treatment

Rectal vault empty
│
Bisocodyl 2–4 QD
May add MOM 30 cc QD

Goal: Bowel movement every 48 hours	Address Environment: *Privacy* *Gastrocolec reflex* *Assistance with feeding and hydration*
Increased risk of impaction if interval between bowel movements > 48 hours	*Access to toilet* *Maximize activity*

Constipation

Selected Readings

Overview

Ross, D. D. and C. S. Alexander. "Management of Common Symptoms in Terminally Ill Patients; Part II. Constipation, Delirium, and Dyspnea." [Review] [39 refs]. *American Family Physician* 15; 64 (2001): 1019–1026.

Fallon, M. and B. O'Neill. "ABC of Palliative Care: Constipation and Diarrhea." *British Medical Journal* 315 (1997): 1293–1296.

Sykes, N. P. "Constipation." In *Principles and Practice of Supportive Oncology,* edited by A. M. Berger, R. K. Portenoy, and D. E. Weissman. New York: Lippincott Williams & Wilkins Healthcare 5 (2002): 1–13.

Constipation in Advanced Cancer

Mancini, I. L., J. Hanson, C. M. Neumann, and E. D. Bruera: "Opioid Type and Other Clinical Predictors of Laxative Dose in Advanced Cancer Patients: A Retrospective Study." *Journal of Palliative Medicine* 3 (2000): 49–56.

McMillan, S. C. "Presence and Severity of Constipation in Hospice Patients with Advanced Cancer." *American Journal of Hospice and Palliative Care* 19 (2002): 426–430.

1.4 Dyspnea

Key Points

1. Dyspnea is the subjective sense of breathlessness or smothering.
    Patients can self-report the severity of their dyspnea using a scale similar to the pain scale. Hypoxia and dyspnea are not always concordant; patients with hypoxia may or may not have dyspnea. Dyspnea is reported by over half of patients at Life's End.

2. Dyspnea may have multiple causes.
    Palliative care does not exclude the search for and treatment of the underlying causes of dyspnea. Palliative care recognizes that the causes of the dyspnea may not be responsive to treatment or that the burden of treatment may outweigh the benefit.

3. Oxygen alone often does not relieve dyspnea.
    Oxygen is a potent symbol of medical care. However, patients routinely can neither tolerate, nor have available in the home, more than 2–5 L of Oxygen by nasal prong. Oxygen alone is usually not adequate treatment to relieve chronic dyspnea.

4. Low-dose opioids can often safely relieve symptoms of dyspnea.
    Low doses of short-acting oral opioids often can reduce dyspnea without sedation or respiratory depression.

5. Dyspnea causes chronic anxiety, which may respond to low-dose benzodiazepines.

6. Dyspnea often responds to non-pharmacological interventions better than to oxygen.
    Many patients find that a fan blowing cool air on the face is more effective for the relief of dyspnea than a 100% non-rebreather mask.

Dyspnea

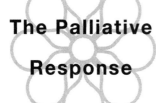

The Palliative Response

The Experience of Dyspnea

- Shortness of breath
- Breathlessness
- Smothering feeling
- Suffocation
- Present at rest
- Worsened by activity

Diagnosing Dyspnea

- Self-report is the key
  To detecting dyspnea
  To appreciating the severity of dyspnea
- Use analog scale to help people self-report severity of shortness of breath
  Now?
  At the worst?
  At the best?
  After treatment?

Diagnosing Dyspnea

- Prevalence may be greater in patients with life-threatening illness
  COPD
  CHF
  Lung cancer
- Blood gas, oxygen saturation, and respiratory rate do not substitute for patient's self-assessment and report of dyspnea

Fix It versus *Treat It*
Paradigm

- Look for reversible causes
- Help patients, families, and colleagues consider the burden of treatment of the underlying cause versus the benefit of treatment

Fix It versus *Treat It*
Paradigm

- Treat dyspnea as a symptom while looking for a reversible cause
- The cause of the dyspnea may take some time to improve
- Often dyspnea does not have a reversible cause, yet patients do not have to suffer unrelieved dyspnea for the remainder of life

Potentially Reversible
Causes of Dyspnea

- Pneumonia and bronchitis
- Pulmonary edema
- Tumor and pleural effusions
- Bronchospasm
- Airway obstruction
- COPD
- Asthma
- Thick secretions

Potentially Reversible
Causes of Dyspnea

- Anxiety
- Pulmonary embolism
- Anemia
- Metabolic disturbance
- Hypoxemia
- Family and practical issues
- Environmental problems

Benefit versus Burden
of Treatment

- It is always important to consider causes of dyspnea
- However, before deciding the extent of evaluation beyond history and physical, begin to weigh benefit versus burden of disease-modifying treatment.

Symptomatic Management
Oxygen

- Oxygen is a potent symbol of medical care
- Try to avoid mask
  Causes discomfort from sense of smothering
  Involves unpleasant accumulation of mucus and moisture
  Interferes with communication and oral intake

Symptomatic Management
Oxygen

- Use humidifier if using nasal prong
- Most people will not tolerate more than 2 l/m
- Be guided by patient comfort, not by oxygen saturation
- Home oxygen is usually provided by a concentrator, which cannot provide more than 5 l/m
- A fan or air conditioner may provide the same level of comfort

Symptomatic Management
Opioids

- Opioids are the most effective treatment for unrelieved dyspnea
- Central and peripheral effects
- Begin with small doses of short-acting opioids
- MS 5mg or Oxycodone 5mg orally q4 hours *Offer/May Refuse* is often a good starting point
- Use analog scale as in pain management to monitor effect

Symptomatic Management
Opioids

- Physicians are afraid people will stop breathing
- It may reassure wary colleagues of the safety of this approach to order *Give if respiratory rate of greater than 20/m*, since relief of dyspnea may not be related to decrease in rate

Symptomatic Management
Nonpharmacological

- Fan
- Keep environment cool, but avoid chilling patient
- Consider cool foods
- Reposition patient; allow to sit up in bed or chair
- Avoid environmental irritants
- Avoid claustrophobic settings
- Have a plan for the next episode of dyspnea to give patient and family sense of control

Symptomatic Management
Anxiolyics

- Anxiety may be a component for patients suffering with dyspnea
- Lorazepam (Ativan) is safe to combine with opioids for dyspnea

  0.5–1mg prn q2 hours may be helpful

  Some patients may benefit from scheduled doses

Dyspnea Review

- Dyspnea is common in patients referred to palliative care
- Dyspnea is also common in the general patient population
- Dyspnea can be effectively controlled in most patients whether or not referred to palliative care
- Visual analog scale is the best tool for assessing dyspnea and monitoring effectiveness of its treatment

Dyspnea

Selected Readings

Overview of Dyspnea Treatment

Shaiova, L. A. "Management of Dyspnea in Patients with Advanced Cancer." In *Principles and Practice of Supportive Oncology* edited by A. M. Berger, R. K. Portenoy, and D. E. Weissman. New York: Lipincott Williams & Wilkins Healthcare 2 (1999): 1–11.

Thomas, J. R. and C. F. Von Gunten. "Treatment of Dyspnea in Cancer Patients." *Oncology* 16 (2002): 745–750.

Zeppetella, G. "The Palliation of Dyspnea in Terminal Disease." *American Journal of Hospice and Palliative Care* Nov/Dec (1998): 322–330.

Oral Morphine as Symptomatic Treatment

Boyd, K. J. and M. Kelly. "Oral Morphine as Symptomatic Treatment of Dyspnea in Patients with Advanced Cancer." *Palliative Medicine* 11 (1997): 277–281.

Management of Dyspnea and Cough

Dudgeon, D. J. and S. Rosenthal. "Management of Dyspnea and Cough in Patients with Cancer." *Hematology/Oncology Clinics of North America* 10 (1996): 157–171.

1.5 Insomnia

Key Points

1. Insomnia manifests as nonrefreshing sleep, difficulty falling asleep or maintaining sleep, or early morning awakening. It causes daytime sleepiness and poor concentration, diminished coping and QOL, and exhaustion in family and caregivers.

2. Insomnia is common and increases with age or illness.

     About 50% of advanced cancer patients report insomnia, and about 75% of patients admitted to a palliative-care unit require hypnotic medication.

3. Assessment includes differential diagnosis that considers treatment or medication side effects, poor sleep environment, mental disorders, primary sleep disorders, physical symptoms, and the effect of substances or substance withdrawal.

     Effects of sleep environment can include uncomfortable bed, lights, noise, odors, being awakened for vital signs or blood draws, blood transfusion, and monitoring devices or alarms. Substance effects many include use of coffee, tobacco, or caffeine, or withdrawal from alcohol or benzodiazepines. Medications requiring evaluation include steroids, albuterol, theophyline, and stimulants.

4. The physician assesses for insomnia by questions about its presence, chronicity, or acuteness, factors associated with sleep difficulties and efforts to address them, as well as inquiries about differential diagnoses.

5. Management of insomnia includes improving symptom control and identifying and treating contributory factors.

     Delirium, common at Life's End, may be mistaken for insomnia, and some insomnia medications can worsen delirium. The physician can stop unnecessary medications and move steroids and stimulants to morning doses. Sleep hygiene interventions include exercising earlier in the day, following a bedtime ritual, practicing relaxation techniques, and restricting use of bed to sleeping.

6. Trazedone is a common regimen based on the anecdotal experience of hospice programs.

     There is not good evidence about the medication most effective for insomnia. The Trazedone dose may vary from 25–100mg q hs.

Insomnia

The Palliative Response

What Is Insomnia?

- Manifestations
  Nonrefreshing sleep
  Difficulty falling asleep
  Early morning awakening
  Difficulty maintaining sleep

- Symptoms
  Daytime sleepiness
  Daytime lack of concentration

Prevalence

- Common in the population
- Increases with age or illness
  Advanced cancer
  ~ 50% of patients report insomnia Palliative Care patients
  ~75% of patients admitted to a palliative-care unit require a hypnotic medicine

Cycle

- Etiology
  Pain and other symptoms lead to insomnia
- Sequelae
  Insomnia exacerbates other symptoms and makes them harder to bear
- Effects
  Diminishes coping capacity
  Lowers reported QOL
  Exhausts family and caregivers

Differential Diagnosis

- Treatment side effects
  Diarrhea, nausea, instrumentation
  Chemotherapy induced mucositis, pain
- Poor sleep environment
  Uncomfortable bed, lights, noise, odors
  Awakened for vital signs, blood draws, etc.
  Blood transfusion
  Monitoring devices and alarms

Differential Diagnosis

- Mental disorders
  Depression, delirium, anxiety
- Substances
  Coffee, tobacco, caffeine
- Withdrawal from substances
  Alcohol, benzodiazepines, other drugs
- Medications
  Steroids, albuterol, theophyline, stimulants

Differential Diagnosis

- Primary sleep disorder
  Sleep apnea
  Restless legs syndrome

- Physical symptoms
  Pain, dyspnea, cough
  Diarrhea, nausea, pruritis

Assessment

- Do you experience insomnia?
- Chronic problem or new with this illness?
- What do you think makes it hard to sleep?
- What works and doesn't work to help?
- Depression or anxiety causing problems?
- Stimulants, like coffee or alcohol, before sleep?

Management of Insomnia

- Improve control of pain or other symptoms

- Identify and treat depression

- Identify and treat delirium
  Common at Life's End
  May be mistaken for insomnia
  Worsened by some insomnia medications

Management of Insomnia

- Support treatment for known primary sleep disorder
  E.g., CPAP for sleep apnea

- Review medications
  Stop unneeded medicines
  Administer steroids/stimulants in morning
  Counsel about caffeine, alcohol, tobacco

Management of Insomnia
Sleeping Environment

- Comfortable bed and position
- Appropriate lighting and noise level (some people need white noise)
- Reduce interruptions such as vital signs, medicine, blood draws, transfusions
- Reduce instrumentation and monitors with alarms

Management of Insomnia
Sleep Hygiene

- Exercise earlier in day
- Establish bedtime ritual
- Employ relaxation techniques
- Restrict use of bed
  Bed is for sleeping
  If unable to sleep, get out of bed

Medications for Sleep
Trazedone

- Lack of good evidence about most effective medication for insomnia

- Trazedone 25–100mg q hs
  Has become a common regimen
  Problems with other medications
  Positive anecdotal experience of hospice programs

Medications for Sleep
Benzodiazepine Hypnotic

- Meant for short-term use (2 weeks or less)
- Tolerance develops rapidly
- May contribute to delirium
- Problems of withdrawal
- Short-acting forms—wake up in night
- Long-acting forms—daytime grogginess

Medications for Sleep
GABA/BZD Agents

- Examples
  Zalepion (Sonata)
  Zolpidem (Ambien)

- Comparison with benzodiazepine
  Act at same site
  Same problems and precautions
  Cost significantly more without clear benefit

Medications for Sleep
Antidepressants

- Good choice if someone is depressed
- Trazedone
  Has become antidepressant of choice
  Fewer side effects
- Doxipen and Imipramine
  More sedating
- Side Effects
  Constipation
  Dry mouth
  Orthostatis

Medications for Sleep
Antihistamines

- Usually not drug of choice
  Short-term effect
  Numerous interactions with other medications
  May contribute to delirium
- Benadryl is in many over-the-counter sleep aids
- Herbal or natural remedies untested

Review of Insomnia

- Assessment
  Often multifactorial
  Reassess frequently
- Treatment
  Treat underlying causes if possible
  Use hypnotic medications if needed
- Goals of Care
  Restful sleep
  Improved QOL and daytime functioning

Selected Readings

Savard, J. and C. Morin. "Insomnia in the Context of Cancer: A Review of a Neglected Problem." *Journal of Clinical Oncology* 19 (2001): 14.

1.6 Nausea and Vomiting

Key Points

1. Nausea is a source of distress even if vomiting does not occur.
   Nausea is a complex symptom that may lead to vomiting by activation of the vomiting center and retroperistalsis. There are four major sources of input into the vomiting center. Patients often have more than one source of input.

2. Nausea may be due to fear and anxiety.
   Fear and anxiety can lead to anticipatory nausea.

3. Nausea may be due to increased intracranial pressure.
   Pressure may be due to metastatic or primary tumor, intracerebral bleed or trauma, hydrocephalus, or infection.

4. Nausea may be due to vestibular dysfunction.
   Vertigo may be due to inner-ear infection, sinus congestion, primary vertigo, or hyponatremia.

5. Nausea may be due to the action of drugs, uremia, hypercalcemia, or acidosis upon the chemoreceptor trigger zone.
   Multiple medications and metabolic disturbances can affect the chemoreceptor trigger zone. A careful review of medications is indicated. However, if individual needs the opioid for pain and dyspnea control, it is better to treat the nausea than to stop the opioid.

6. Nausea may be due to GI disorders such as constipation, obstruction, gastroparesis, gastritis, metastatic disease, hepatomegaly, or ascites.
   Prevention of constipation and use of a prokinetic like metochlopromide are key to managing this source of nausea.

Nausea and Vomiting

The Palliative Response

Nausea

- The unpleasant feeling that there is a need to vomit

- A source of distress even if vomiting does not occur

- Accompanied by tachycardia, increased salivation, pallor, and sweating

Retching and Vomiting

- Retching

  Spasmodic contractions of the diaphragm and abdominal muscle

  May lead to vomiting

  May persist after the stomach has emptied

- Vomiting

  Expulsion of the gastric content through the mouth

The Vomiting Center

- Tractus solitarus, reticular formation in the medulla
- Parasympathetic motor efferents

  Contraction of pylorsis

  Reduction of lower esophogeal sphincter (LES)

  Contraction of stomach

- Retroperistalsis

Input
Into the Vomiting Center

- Fear and anxiety

  May cause anticipatory nausea

- Increased intracranial pressure

  Metastatic tumor

  Primary tumor

  Intracerebral bleed/trauma

  Hydrocephalus

  Infection

Treatmen

- Fear and anxiety

  Lorazepam: 1mg q6–8 hours

  Counseling

- Increased intracranial pressure

  Dexamethasone: 4–10mg q6

  Mannitol infusion (short-term bridge to definitive treatment)

  Radiation therapy

  Neurosurgery

Input
Into the Vomiting Center

- Vestibular dysfunction (Vertigo)

  Causes: *Inner ear infection*
  Sinus congestion
  Primary vertigo
  Hyponatremia

  1st line treatment:
  Antihistamines
  Meclizine

  2nd line treatment:
  Anticholinergic
  Scopolamine
  Hyoscine

Input
Into the Vomiting Center

- Chemoreceptor trigger zone

  Drugs
  Opioids
  Digoxin
  Antibiotics
  Cytotoxics
  Anticonvulsants

  Uremia

  Hypercalcemia

  Acidosis

Input
Into the Vomiting Center

- Chemoreceptor trigger zone

  1st line treatment:
  Dopamine antagonist
  Haloperidol
  Prochlorperazine
  Metoclopramide

  2nd line treatment:
  5HT3 antagonist ondanstron

  Nonspecific
  Dexamethasone

Input
Into the Vomiting Center

- GI disorders
  Constipation
  GI obstruction
  Gastroparesis
  Gastritis (NSAID)
  Metastatic disease
  Hepatomegaly
  Ascites

Treatment
GI Disorders

- Relieve constipation
- Relieve obstruction
- Review medications

Treatment
GI Disorders

- H2 blockers or PPI
- 1st line treatment:
  Metoclopramide
- Consider
  5HT3
  Dexamethasone
  Bowel rest

Treatment Plan

- Relaxing and nonstressful environment
- Medication after meals, except for anti-emetics
- Mouth care and topical anti-fungal prn
- Remove sources of offensive odors
- Small portions, frequent meals
- Monitor for constipation or bladder distention

Treatment Plan

- Dexamethasone as a non-specific anti-inflammatory
- Cannabinoids (Marijuana or Marinol)
- Some new atypical anti-depressants (Rimeron)
- When all else fails, go back to beginning
- If mechanical obstruction, may benefit from octratide (see plan of care for GI obstruction)

Input into Vomiting Center

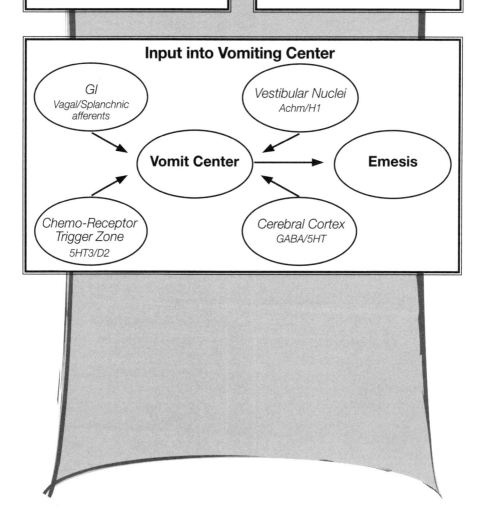

Nausea and Vomiting

Selected Readings

Overview

Baines, M. J. "ABC of Palliative Care: Nausea, Vomiting, and Intestinal Obstruction." *British Medical Journal* 315 (1997): 1148–1150.

Management

Rousseau, P. "Nonpain Symptom Management in Terminal Care." *Clinics in Geriatric Medicine: Care of the Terminally Ill Patient.* 0749–0690/ 96: 315–326.

1.7 Feeding by Mouth

Key Points

1. It is important to create a setting conducive to feeding by mouth.

2. Special eating procedures are helpful for patients with asthenia or neuromuscular disorders.

3. Encourage oral hygiene, treat for infection, and order dental work as needed. Treat taste disorders by addressing underlying disease and the symptom of bad taste.

4. Treat dry mouth from radiation with saliva substitute and frequent sips of water.
   When dry mouth is a side effect of medication, substitute drugs or reduce dosage if possible. Address dry mouth in the last hours of life by increasing liquids by mouth or involving family in mouth care.

5. Suspect and assess for Oral Candidiasis (Thrush) as cause of problems with eating. Viral infections and cold sores are usually caused by herpetic infection.

6. To manage Reflux Esophagitis, keep patient upright, serve small meals, and use prokinetic, H2 blockers, and proton pump inhibitors if needed.

7. Mucositis is a somatic type of pain that usually responds to opioid therapy. Treat Mucositis with oral lavage with soda water, "Magic/ Miracle Mouthwash" or Viscous Xylocaine.

8. Difficulty with eating is common at Life's End, causes significant distress, and is often multifactorial. Careful and thoughtful evaluation can relieve suffering, improve Quality of Life, and increase oral intake in the majority of patients.

Feeding by Mouth

The Palliative Response

The Setting

- Environment—calm and unhurried
- Posture —upright (chair is preferable)
  Edge of bed preferable to in bed, but unstable
- Assistance from family or nursing staff
  Free nursing time by eliminating activities unnecessary at Life's End (e.g., frequent vital signs)
- Role of occupational therapy
  Special aids (sipper cups/wide-grip utensils)
  Straws increase risk of aspiration

Asthenia or Neuromuscular Disorders
Preparation for Eating

Posture
- Upright position
- Stabilize the head

Meal
- Small frequent meals
- Bite-sized pieces, soft pureed food
- Moisten food with gravy or sauces
- Patients prefer soft and cool foods
- Supplements such as Ensure may be helpful, especially for elderly who prefer sweet foods

Asthenia or Neuromuscular Disorders
Safety Precautions

Eating
- Encourage small sips to clear mouth
- Remind patients to chew thoroughly
- Meal may take 30–45 minutes

Post-Meal Precaution
- Reduce risk of reflux by encouraging upright position for 15–30 minutes after eating

Dentures

Hygiene
- Assist patient with cleaning and use

Proper Fit
- May need adhesive
- May need to be refitted or replaced

Personal Preference
- Some patients prefer to wear dentures
- Others choose to stop wearing

Oral Hygiene

Cleanliness
- Encourage and assist with brushing and flossing 2–3 times day

Preventing Infection
- Antibiotics for periodontal disease

Dental Intervention
- Dental work or extraction if indicated
- Fluoride treatment as needed in special cases

Taste Disorders

Treat Underlying Disorder
- Sinusitis or other infections
- Gastric reflux
- Excessive sputum

Treat Symptom of Bad Taste
- Supplements, especially zinc, may provide relief
- Review medications that may taste bad

Dry Mouth
from Radiation

Medical Treatment
- Saliva substitute every 1–2 hours
- Pilocarpine 5mg q8 hours
  Rarely used
  May cause diarrhea or problems with secretions

Other Interventions
- Usually frequent sips of water sufficient
- Sipper cup or sports bottle easier for patient than straws

Dry Mouth
from Medication

- Seek to avoid side effect of dry mouth
- Substitute drug if possible
  Trazedone instead of amitriptyline for insomnia
- Reduce dosage if possible

Dry Mouth
in Last Hours of Life

- Increase liquids by mouth
  Ice chips
  Popsicles
  Flavored ices
- Mouth care may be more effective and can involve family in care
  Assisted sips
  Moistened sponge stick
  Lip balm
  Antifungal creams for celosis

Oral Candidiasis (Thrush)

Assessment
- Always suspect this infection as cause of problems with eating

Treatment
- Nystatin suspension swish and swallow
- Fluconazole (Diflucan)
  100mg daily for 10–14 days
  More expensive
  Easier and more quickly effective

Viral Infections: Cold Sores

Etiology
- Usually caused by herpetic infection

Treatment
- Consider Acylovir (Zovirax)
- Consider other antiviral treatment in cases of resistance and other special factors

Reflux Esophagitis
Practical Considerations

- Small meals
- Keep patient upright after meals

Medical management
- May need prokinetic such as metoclopromide
- Manage constipation
- H2 blockers
- Proton pump inhibitors

Mucositis
Oral Lavage with Soda Water

Procedure
- Baking soda (sodium bicarbonate)
  15 grams to a liter of water
- Swish and spit
- Keep at bedside for patient to use as needed

Advantage
- Helps cleanse mouth of dead tissue and debris
- Does not burn

Mucositis
Magic/Miracle Mouthwash

- Consult pharmacy about preparation
  Combination of medications
  May contain diphenhydramine, viscous xylocaine, Maalox, nystatin, tetracycline
- Order bottle to bedside for use by patient as needed
- Alternate with soda-wash rinse

Mucositis
Viscous Xylocaine

Dosage
- 2% 5ml every 4 hours as needed

Preparation
- Flavor or dilute to lessen its bad taste

Timing
- Sometimes used before meals
- May make it harder to swallow— changes sensation in mouth

Mucositis
Overview

- A somatic type of pain
- Opioid therapy
  Patients can usually benefit and respond
  May need to give opioid parentrally in severe cases
- Indications for Thalidomide 200mg daily
  Severe mucosal damage
  Ulceration not responding to other treatments
  Drug of last choice (may wish to consult first)

Difficulty with Eating

Prevalence
- Common in patients

Suffering
- Causes significant distress

Etiology
- Often multifactorial

Hope
- Careful and thoughtful evaluation can relieve suffering, improve Quality of Life, and increase oral intake

Feeding by Mouth

Selected Readings

Nutrition and Hydration: A Sociological Analysis

McInerney, F. "Provision of Food and Fluids in Terminal Care: A Sociological Analysis." *Social Science and Medicine* 34: 1271–1276.

Prevention of Tube Feeding

Volicer, L. "Strategies for Prevention of Tube Feeding in Advanced Dementia." *Quarterly Newsletter of the American Academy of Hospice and Palliative Medicine* 1 (2001): 16–18.

Treatment of Common Oral Conditions

Bottomley, W. K. and S. W. Rosenberg eds. *Clinician's Guide to Treatment of Common Oral Conditions*. The American Academy of Oral Medicine: 1973; Fall.

1.8 Hydration

Key Points

1. Appetite and oral intake usually decline in the final days of life to a few sips or bites. Goals of hydration are to maintain function, improve Quality of Life, improve delirium, help satisfy sense of thirst and hunger, and engage family and friends in care.

2. Signs and symptoms of dehydration are more important than lab tests.

3. Benefits of <u>oral hydration</u> include low technology, minimal risk, ease of home use, fostering of human contact and pleasure, and low risk of causing fluid overload.
   Foster hydration with pleasant liquids, drinking aids and companionship/assistance at meals. Replete electrolytes naturally with sports drinks and tomato-based juices; hydrate naturally with sips of fluid. Two tablespoons of fluid four times in an hour equals 120ml of fluid. An IV at the rate of 75cc/hr takes 5 hours to infuse fluids equivalent to a canned drink (355 ml).

4. The burdens of <u>enteral feeding (NG/PEG)</u> usually outweigh the benefits.
   NG/PEG tube feeding at Life's End causes the discomfort of invasive procedures and restraints and the risk of aspiration, infections, nausea, diarrhea, distention, edema, and pulmonary congestion.

5. <u>Hypodermoclysis</u> offers a simple technique of administration of subcutaneous fluids, but policies and staff training in most clinical settings do not support its use.
   Burdens include possibility of dislodging needle, necessity of restraints, pain and swelling at site, risk of fluid overload, and cost of treatment.

6. <u>Parenteral intravenous administration</u> of fluids can be difficult and painful. Its use risks infections, restraints and fluid overload and creates a barrier to home care.

7. Key considerations in palliative hydration include evaluating burdens and benefits in the context of Goals of Care, seeking reversible cause, trying oral route, and observing for safety if an invasive route is indicated as a bridge to oral hydration.

Hydration

The Palliative Response

Goals of Hydration

- Help maintain function
- Improve Quality of Life
- May improve delirium
- Help satisfy subjective sensation of thirst and hunger
- Engage family and friends in care

Appetite and Oral Intake
at Life's End

- Status

  Declines in most patients

  People may take only few sips or bites in last days of life

- Typical Clinical Response

  Most hospital and nursing home patients have feeding tubes and/or IV's at time of death

Indications for Hydration

- Reversible Process (e.g., constipation)

- Treatable Infection (e.g., thrush)

- Temporary Insult

Burdens
Enteral and Perenteral Fluids

- Invasive procedures
- Pain and distress
- Edema and pulmonary congestion
- Provide little comfort
- Burden adds to suffering
- Burden often outweighs benefit

Diagnostic and Treatment
Considerations

Diagnosis
- Signs and symptoms more important than lab tests

  Skin tenting

  Concentrated urine with decline in output

  Postural symptoms

  Dry mouth

Treatment
- Look for reversible causes of decline
- Easier to manage early than late
- Consider appetite stimulant

Complication
Enteral and Parenteral Fluids

- Edema (third-spacing of fluids)

  Indicates intravascular fluid depletion rather than pure dehydration

  Often worsened by E/P fluids

- Often worsen pulmonary congestion

- Often lead to dyspnea without other benefits

Typical Concerns
Patients and Caregivers

- Dependence on others to be fed

- Loss of appetite

- Weight loss

- Loss of food as symbol of love

Fostering Patient Control

Some persons refuse food or fluid as way of having control.

- Foster control and good decisions by providing accurate information
- Provide patient-directed diet
- Feature foods easily swallowed/digested

Dehydration

- Items for dry mouth and sense of thirst

  Ice chips

  Ice cream, puddings

  Frozen popsicles
- Drinking aids

  Sipper cups, wide grips

  "Thick-it" for fluids assists with swallowing
- Companionship and assistance at meals

Ideas for Oral Hydration

- Replete electrolytes

  Sports drinks

  Tomato-based juices for sodium

- Hydrate with sips

  Two tablespoons of fluid four times in an hour equals 120ml of fluid

  Encourage families to offer sips with each TV commercial

  An IV at rate of 75cc/hr takes 5 hours to infuse fluids equivalent to a canned drink (355ml)

Oral Hydration
Benefit Review

- Low technology
- Minimal risk
- Effectively administered at home
- Encourages human contact
- Can be pleasurable for patient
- Less risk of causing fluid overload

Enteral (NG/PEG)
Tube-Feeding at Life's End

- No evidence of benefit

  Causes patient discomfort

  Increases use of restraints

- Sometimes Goals of Care dictate a trial

  (e.g., patient with esophageal cancer and PEG tube undergoing palliative radiation to resolve esophageal obstruction)

  Ask: Is tube-feeding a bridge to resuming oral intake?

Enteral Feedings
Benefits
- Increase mental alertness
- Reduce family anxiety
- Potentially prolong life for special event

Burdens
- Risk of aspiration
- Potential for infections
- Diarrhea and distention
- Nausea
- Invasive procedures
- Restraints

Hypodermoclysis
Subcutaneous Fluids
(30–50cc/hr of D5 ½ normal saline)

Advantages
- Simple technology for home use

Disadvantages
- Hospitals/nursing homes often not prepared
- Needle may still come dislodged
- Pain and swelling at site
- Some risk of fluid overload
- May still need restraints
- Cost of treatment

Ask: Is this a bridge to resuming oral intake?

Parenteral Feeding
Intravenous Fluids

Disadvantages
- Invasive
- Can be difficult and painful to insert IV
- Risk of infections
- Use of restraints
- Risk of fluid overload
- Sometimes seen as barrier to home care

Parenteral
Intravenous Fluids
Considerations

- Goals of Care

  Is this a bridge to resuming oral intake?

- Consider time trial (2 liters over 8 hours)

  Stop IV fluids if not helpful

  Parenteral fluids may blunt thirst and hunger

  Some patients resume oral intake when fluids discontinued

- Avoid KVO fluids

Hydration
The Palliative Response

- Try the oral route
- Seek reversible cause of decreased oral intake
- Balance burden against benefit of perenteral and enteral hydration
- Consider Goals of Care
- If using a more invasive route

  Consider a time trial

  Observe carefully to maintain safety and prevent iatrogenic harm

Hydration

Selected Readings

Nutrition and Hydration: Appropriate Use

McCann, R. M., W. J. Hall, and A. Groth-Juncker. "Comfort Care for Terminally Ill Patients: the Appropriate Use of Nutrition and Hydration." *Journal of the American Medical Association* 272 (1994): 1263–1266.

Onwuteaka-Phillipsen B. D., H. R. Pasman, A. Kruit, A. van der Heide, M. W. Ribbe, and G. van der Wal: "Withholding or Withdrawing Artificial Administration of Food and Fluids in Nursing-Home Patients." *Age and Ageing* 30 (2001): 459–465.

—— Comment in: *Age and Ageing* (2001): 436–438.

Nutrition and Hydration: A Sociological Analysis

McInerney, F. "Provision of Food and Fluids in Terminal Care: A Sociological Analysis." *Social Science and Medicine* 34: 1271–1276.

Treatment of Common Oral Conditions

Bottomley, W. K. and S. W. Rosenberg eds. *Clinician's Guide to Treatment of Common Oral Conditions.* The American Academy of Oral Medicine, 1973; Fall.

1.9 Intestinal Obstruction

Key Points

1. Intestinal obstruction is associated with ovarian and colorectal cancers (often a late manifestation) and is common with abdominal and pelvic primary tumors.

   Obstruction may be partial or complete, intermittent or persistent, have single versus multiple sites, and present in the small or large bowel.

2. Surgery is the best palliative treatment if possible.

   Co-morbid illness or progression of disease may make non-surgical management preferable.

3. Goals of Care in managing intestinal obstructions are relief of pain, nausea, and vomiting; avoidance of NG tube; and support of patient and family in an emotionally charged situation.

   Situation is charged because of patient's inability to eat and imminent death often within a few days to no more than a few weeks.

4. Consider subcutaneous, sublingual, topical, intravenous, or rectal routes for administration of medication. Oral route is not reliable.

   Usually choose morphine for pain control. Use sublingual or subcutaneous route, titrate dose to comfort, use small and frequent dosing schedule, or use pump with both continuous and PCA.

5. Octreotide puts the intestines at rest.

   Stops peristalsis against site of obstruction, reduces gastric secretions, increases electrolyte and fluid re-absorption, and often substantially reduces nausea and vomiting.

6. Antiemetics may be helpful. Patient may still vomit several times a day, but most prefer this to NG tube placement.

   Antiemetics include dopamine antagonist, haloperidol 1 SQ q6 (less sedating), chlorpromazine 25mg q6 PR (more sedating, less acceptable), and Lorazepam 1–2mg SQ q6 (if patient is anxious and sedation is welcomed).

7. Most patients will moderate oral intake on their own. It is not necessary to make patients completely NPO. Offer ice chips, sherbet, or juice.

Intestinal Obstruction

The Palliative Response

Diagnostic Considerations

- Etiology
  Ovarian cancer— late manifestation
  Colorectal cancers—late manifestation
  Abdominal tumors
  Pelvic primary tumors

- Distinctions
  Partial versus complete
  Intermittent versus persistent
  Single versus multiple sites
  Small versus large bowel

Management

- Surgical
  Best palliative treatment, if possible
  Not possible in some patients

- Nonsurgical
  Co-morbid illness may make it preferable
  Progression of disease may make it preferable

Good Prognostic Factors for Surgery

- Large-bowel obstruction treated with diverting colostomy
- Single site of obstruction
- Absence of ascites
- Good preoperative performance status

Poor Prognostic Factors for Surgery

- Proximal gastric obstruction or SBO
- Ascites
- Multiple sites of obstruction
- Diffuse peritoneal carcinomatosis
- Previous surgery and radiation treatment
- Poor performance and nutritional status
- Significant distant metastatic disease

Placing Stents by Endoscopy

- Esophageal obstruction
- Rectal obstruction
- Less effective in other sites
- Sometimes well tolerated but can lead to perforation, obstruction, and pain
- Usually only a temporary solution

NG or Venting Gastrostomy

- Most helpful in more proximal obstruction
- Decompresses the stomach but NG tube not tolerated long-term
- Venting gastrostomy may be more acceptable for longer term
- Rarely used due to generally poor condition of patients

Goals of Care

- Relief of pain
- Relief of nausea and vomiting
- Avoidance of the NG tube
- Support of patient and family as unit
  Emotionally charged situation
  Inability to eat
  Imminent death, often within a few days to few weeks

Route of Medication

- Oral route not reliable

- Alternatives to oral route
  Subcutaneous
  Sublingual
  Topical
  Intravenous
  Rectal

Pain Management

Usually morphine

- Sublingual or subcutaneous route
- Titrate dose to comfort
- Usually best to use small, frequent dosing schedule
- Pumps with both continuous and PCA are often best choice

Dexamethasone

40mg IV QD for 4 days

- Consider in most patients
- May result in reduction of edema around the site of obstruction and in temporary relief of obstruction
- May enable to resume oral medications including dexamethosone
- If not effective, can discontinue

Octreotide

0.1–2mg SQ q8 hours

- Puts bowel to rest and stops peristalsis against site of obstruction
- Reduces gastric secretions
- Increases electrolyte and fluid re-absorption
- Often substantially reduces nausea and vomiting

Antisecretory Drugs

- Reduce saliva and secretions
  Produce up to 2 liters a day
  If obstructed, patient must vomit back up
- Scopolamine topically
- Glycopyrrolate 0.1–2mg SQ q8 hours
- H2 blockade or proton-pump inhibitors
  May reduce gastric acid secretions

Antiemetics

- Metocholopramide (Reglan)
  A prokinetic—not appropriate if obstruction complete
  May be helpful in partial obstruction
  Time trial—stop if colic worsens
- Dopamine antagonist
  Haloperidol 1 SQ q6 is less sedating
  Chlopromazine 25mg q6 PR is more sedating (less acceptable)
- Lorazepam 1–2mg SQ q6
  If patient is anxious and sedation is welcomed

Medical Management

- Outcome
  These regimens relieve symptoms satisfactorily in most patients
  Patient may still vomit several times a day but usually prefers this to NG tube placement

- Oral Intake
  Offer ice chips, sherbet, or juice
  Most patients will moderate oral intake
  Not necessary or kind to make completely NPO

Total Parenteral Nutrition (TPN)

- Usually not recommended
- May have deleterious effects
- Problems with infections
- Very select patient population may benefit

Hydration

- Assess burden versus benefit
  Appropriate only for selected patients
  May be difficult to maintain IV site
  Problems with fluid overload

- Hypodermoclysis
  Hydration via the subcutaneous route
  May be helpful in selected patients

Management

- Selection of treatment
  No comparative studies to determine best treatment in management of obstruction
- Assess benefit and burden daily
- Adjust medication
  Maximize control of symptoms
  Support patient and family

Selected Readings

Overview

Muir, J. C. "Malignant Bowel Obstruction." In *Principles and Practice of Supportive Oncology* edited by A. M. Berger, R. K. Portenoy, and D. E. Weissman. New York: Lipincott Williams & Wilkins Healthcare 2 (1999): 1–7.

Medical Management

Mystakidou, K., E. Tsilika, O. Kalaidopoulou, K. Chondros, S. Georgaki, and L. Papadimitriou. "Comparision of Octreotide Administration vs Conservative Treatment in the Management of Inoperable Bowel Obstruction in Patients with Far-Advanced Cancer: A Randomized, Double-blind, Controlled Clinical Trial." *Anticancer Research* 22 (2002): 1187–1192.

Von Gunten, C. and J. C. Muir. "Medical Management of Bowel Obstruction. Fast Facts and Concepts #45." *Journal of Palliative Medicine* 5 (2002): 739–741.

1.10 Pain and Pain Control (1)

Key Points

1. Conversion of morphine oral to IV/SQ is 3:1.

   For example, morphine 30mg PO is equal to morphine 10mg IV/SQ.

2. Maximum daily dose of acetaminophen is 4 grams in 24 hours.

   Tylenol #3™ (Codeine 30mg/APAP 325 mg)
   Max in 24 hours equal to 12 tablets

   Percocet™ (Oxycodone 5mg/APAP 325mg)
   Max in 24 hours equal to 12 tablets

   Tylox™ (Oxycodone 5mg/APAP 500mg)
   Max in 24 hours equal to 8 tablets

   Lortab5™ (Hydrocodone 5mg/APAP 500mg)
   Max in 24 hours equal to 8 tablets

3. MSContin or Oromorph should not be prescribed as a PRN medicine or at a frequency of less than 8 hours.

   The half-life of sustained release morphine is 8–12 hours and is not effective for breakthrough pain. It will take five half-lives or about two days to reach a steady state.

4. Fentanyl patch 25mcg/hr, topically exchanged every 3 days, is approximately equivalent to morphine 45mg oral in divided doses over 24 hours.

   The smallest dose of fentanyl is equivalent to 8–10 Percocet or Tylox tablets in a 24-hour period. Opioid-naive patients should not receive fentanyl.

5. Opioid prescriptions self-destruct.

   An opioid prescription expires in three days. Only prescriptions for codeine and hydocodone can be refilled without a new written prescription.

Pain and Pain Control (I and II)

The Palliative Response

Discussion: Ms. Brewster

Ms. Brewster is taking (2) Percocet every 4 hours for bone pain related to osteoporotic spine fracture and collapse

---

Equianalgesic Dose
Morphine-MS Contin

- Ms. Brewster is taking the equivalent of Morphine 90mg in 24 hours

- Calculate the equianalgesic dose for:

A) MS Contin

Equianalgesic Dose
Morphine-Oral MS

- Ms. Brewster is taking the equivalent of Morphine 90mg in 24 hours

- Calculate the equianalgesic dose for:

B) Oral MS immediate release

Equianalgesic Dose
Morphine-Fentanyl Patch

- Ms. Brewster is taking the equivalent of Morphine 90mg in 24 hours

- Calculate the equianalgesic dose for:

C) Fentanyl patch (Duragesic)

Equianalgesic Dose
Morphine-Oral Hydromorphone

- Ms. Brewster is taking the equivalent of Morphine 90mg in 24 hours

- Calculate the equianalgesic dose for:

D) Oral hydromorphone (Dilaudid)

Equianalgesic Dose
Morphine-Oxycontin

- Ms. Brewster is taking the equivalent of Morphine 90mg in 24 hours

- Calculate the equianalgesic dose for:

E) Oxycontin

Equianalgesic Dose
Morphine Patient-Controlled Analgesia (PCA) Pump

- Ms. Brewster is taking the equivalent of Morphine 90mg in 24 hours

- Calculate the equianalgesic dose for:

F) PCA Morphine pump SQ or IV

The Palliative Response

OPIOID EQUIANALGESIC CONVERSION TABLE

(Dosing in mg unless listed)

ORAL	OPIOID AGENT		IV/IM/SQ
30	Morphine (MSC, OSR, Roxanol™)		10
8	Hydromorphone (Dilaudid™)		2
20	Methadone (Dolophine™)		—
300	Meperidine (Demerol™)	100	
30	Oxycodone (Roxicodone™, OxyContin™)		—
4 tabs	Oxycodone 5mg/APAP 325mg (Percocet™)		—
6 tabs	Hydrocodone 5mg/APAP 500mg (Lortab5™)		—
6 tabs	Codeine 30mg/APAP (Tylenol #3™)		—
200+	Codeine		—

FENTANYL PATCH CONVERSION
25mcg/hour topically exchanged every 72 hours is equivalent to the following:
- Morphine 15mg IV or 45mg PO per day
- Hydromorphone 3mg IV or 12mg PO per day
- Percocet ™/ Lortab5™ /Tylenol #3 ™—9 tabs per day

Oxycodone and Acetaminophen

Ms. Brewster is taking (2) Percocet every 4 hours for bone pain related to osteoporotic spine fracture and collapse

- Percocet is oxycodone 5mg/ APAP 325mg
- This is equal to 4 grams of acetaminophen in a 24-hour period
- The maximum daily acetaminophen dose should not exceed 4 grams in 24-hour period

Oxycodone and Morphine

Ms. Brewster is taking (2) Percocet every 4 hours for bone pain related to osteoporotic spine fracture and collapse

- Oxycodone and Morphine are equianalgesic
- 4 Percocet contain 20mg of Oxycodone with APAP and are approximately equivalent to morphine 30mg
- 12 Percocet approximately equal morphine 90mg in divided doses over a 24-hour period

Equianalgesic Dose
Morphine-MS Contin

Ms. Brewster is taking the equivalent of Morphine 90mg in 24 hours

Calculate the equianalgesic dose for:

A) MS Contin

- Comes as MS Contin 15,30,60,100,200mg tablet
- Can be dosed as q8 or q12 hour (not BID or TID)
- Takes 5 half-lives/about 48 hours to reach steady state

Equianalgesic Dose
Morphine-MS Contin

Ms. Brewster is taking the equivalent of Morphine 90mg in 24 hours

Calculate the equianalgesic dose for:

A) MS Contin 30mg q8

- Probably best choice
- Make sure that breakthrough dose of 10–15% is available, particularly until reaches steady state

Equianalgesic Dose
Morphine-Oral MS

Ms. Brewster is taking the equivalent of Morphine 90mg in 24 hours

Calculate the equianalgesic dose for:

B) Oral MS immediate release

- MS elixir 10mg/5ml q2–4
- MS concentrate 20mg/1ml q2
- MSIR 15mg tablets q4

Equianalgesic Dose
Morphine-Oral MS

Ms. Brewster is taking the equivalent of Morphine 90mg in 24 hours

Calculate the equianalgesic dose for:

B) Oral MS immediate release

- MS elixir 10mg/5ml, 7.5ml, or 15mg q4
- MS concentrate 20mg/1ml *Offer* 0.5ml or 10mg q2 *May Refuse*
- MSIR 15mg tablets q4

Fentanyl Patch
(Duragesic)

- Reaches steady state in about 18 hours
- Dose can be escalated every 24 hours
- The medicine is deposited in fat under skin
- Duragesic is expensive
- Some patients have trouble with the patch staying applied
- Must be on central or core body area to be well absorbed

Equianalgesic Dose
Morphine-Fentanyl Patch

Ms. Brewster is taking the equivalent of Morphine 90mg in 24 hours

Calculate the equianalgesic dose for:

C) Fentanyl patch (Duragesic)
   50mcg/top q72 hour

- MS 45mg by mouth, MS 15mg IV in a 24-hour period is equianalgesic to fentanyl 25mcg/hr topically exchanged every 72 hours

Oral Hydromorphone
(Dilaudid)

- Dilaudid 1, 2, 4, or 8mg tablets
- Usually a q4 hour drug
- No sustained release form
- Expensive
- Popular on the street
- Excellent opioid—sometimes fewer side effects than morphine, methadone, or other opioids

Morphine and
Oral Hydromorphone

Ms. Brewster is taking the equivalent of Morphine 90mg in 24 hours

Calculate the equianalgesic dose for:

D) Oral hydromorphone (Diluadid)
   4mg q4 hour by mouth

- Hydromorphone 8mg equianalgesic to MS 30mg/24 hours
- Hydormrophone 24mg equianagesic to MS 90mg/24 hours

Equianalgesic Dose
Morphine-Oxycontin

Ms. Brewster is taking the equivalent of Morphine 90mg in 24 hours

Calculate the equianalgesic dose for:

E) Oxycontin

- Oxycodone and Morphine equianalgesic
- Oxycontin comes as 10, 20, 40mg
- Must be dose q12 hour; do not dose q8 because of longer half-life than Ms Contin
- May increase dose every 48–72 hours

Equianalgesic Dose
Morphine-Oxycontin

Ms. Brewster is taking the equivalent of Morphine 90mg in 24 hours

Calculate the equianalgesic dose for:

E) Oxycontin 40mg po q12 hour with Oxycodone IR 5mg (2)q4 or breakthrough

Equianalgesic Dose
Morphine-IV Morphine

Ms. Brewster is taking the equivalent of Morphine 90mg in 24 hours

Calculate the equianalgesic dose for:

F) <u>IV Morphine</u>

- IV to PO Morphine Conversion is 3:1
- Morphine 90mg PO/24 hours is equal to Morphine 30mg IV/24 hours

Morphine and
PCA Morphine Pump

Ms. Brewster is taking the equivalent of Morphine 90mg in 24 hours

Calculate the equianalgesic dose for:

F) <u>PCA Morphine pump SQ or IV</u>

- MS 1mg/1ml Infuse Continuous at 1mg/hour
- PCA (Patient Control Analgesia) Bolus 1mg q30 minutes

  SQ and IV are equally potent

  SQ does not require maintaining IV site and access

1.11 Pain and Pain Control (II)

Key Points

1. Consider opioid dose escalation if current dose does not control pain.

    For mild to moderate pain, a 25–50% dose escalation is appropriate. For moderate to severe pain, a 50–100% dose escalation is appropriate.

2. Demerol is not recommended for the treatment of pain, due to its toxic metabolites and poor oral absorption.

3. If you expect pain in a patient, consider an Offer/May Refuse order rather than a PRN order for pain medication.

    Delivery of a PRN medication can take over an hour; by then the pain can be quite severe. When the staff offers pain medication at regular intervals, the patient can better control the pain.

4. Sedation, nausea, vomiting, and most opioid side effects are self-limiting and resolve within a few days.

    The physician can anticipate, explain, or treat the side effects to enhance compliance and effective pain control.

5. Anticipate and treat constipation when prescribing opioids, as constipation is not self-limiting.

    Employ a stimulant such as biscodyl or senna to prevent constipation caused by opioids.

6. Pain comes in many forms.

    Somatic pain from tissue injury is the most common type of pain treated with opioids at Life's End. Other kinds of pain (crampy visceral pain, burning and stabbing neuropathic pain) may have some response to opioids, but they benefit more from co-analgesics and adjunctive medicines.

Discussion:
Mr. Norbett

Mr. Norbett, a 72-year-old with metastatic prostate cancer, is admitted with 10/10 back pain that has developed over the last two weeks. He has increased his Percocet use to 2 tablets every 4 hours with minimal effect. He is having difficulty walking because of the pain. The medicine resident is called to the ED to admit him for symptom management and evaluation.

Symptom Management/ Evaluation

The resident writes the following orders:

- MSIR tablets 5mg 2 or 3 tablets po every 4–6 hours prn severe pain
- Tylox 1 or 2 PO every 6 hours mild pain
- MRI of the spine to rule out cord compression

Symptom Management

- The technician sends the patient back to the floor because he is unable to tolerate the MRI and in his agitation has pulled out his IV

- He has received several one-time orders for Demerol 75mgIM

Morphine Dosage

- Calculate the equianalgesic dose of morphine/24hr for the 2 Percocet q4/24hr

- Calculate the minimal and maximal dose of morphine for 24 hours for Mr. Norbett's orders

Morphine Dosage

- Calculate the equianalgesic dose of Morphine/24 hours for the 2 Percocet q4/24 hours
  12 Percocet are approximately equivalent to morphine 90mg PO
- Calculate the minimal and maximal dose of morphine for 24 hours for Mr. Norbett's orders
  Minimal is morphine 40mg/24 hours
  Maximal is morphine 90mg/24 hours

Nursing Response to Opioid Orders

Nursing staff, afraid they will overdose patients and cause them to die, often:

- Pick the weaker of two opioids ordered
- Pick the lower dose
- Pick the longest interval
- Are reluctant to give morphine if Tylox given in the last few hours, even if ineffective

Pain Control

- When pain is poorly controlled
  Use the original daily dose to calculate a new higher dose

- For mild to moderate pain
  Escalate dose by 25–50%

- For moderate to severe pain
  Escalate dose by 50–100%

Safe Escalation of Dosage

- Percocet dose was equivalent to Morphine 90mg PO/24 hours

- Dose escalation of 100% for uncontrolled pain: Morphine 180mg/24 hours

- How to do this safely?

Safe Escalation of Dosage

- MS Elixir (10mg/5ml) 7.5ml or 15mg q2 hours
  Offer/Patient May Refuse

- Morphine PO to IV is a 3:1 ratio

- Morphine 5mg SQ q2 hours
  Offer/Patient May Refuse

Offer/May Refuse Orders
Advantages

- Not PRN

- Patient does not have to wait for nursing staff to check and bring PRN medication, which can take up to an hour

- Patient will not get scheduled dose if sleeping or free of pain

Offer/May Refuse Orders
Implementation

- Use small but frequent doses in dose-finding

- Can switch to long-acting dose based on response

- Can expect response within 4–8 hours

Other Considerations

- Anti-inflammatory medicines are often helpful for bony pain when combined with opioids
- Could use NSAID (e.g., Ibuprofen)
- Could use SAID steroidal anti-inflammatory drugs (e.g., Decadron), which might help with possible cord compression
- Use a large-bowel stimulant (e.g., senna or bisacodyl)

Pain and Pain Control (II)

Selected Readings

Patient's Experience of Pain

Weiss, S. C., L. L. Emanuel, D. L. Fairclough, and E. J. Emanuel. "Understanding the Experience of Pain in Terminally Ill Patients." *The Lancet* 357 (2001): 1311–1315.

Classification of Cancer Pain

Caraceni, A. and Weinstein, S. M. "Classification of Cancer Pain Syndromes." *Oncology* 15 (2001): 1627–1639.

Management of Pain in Palliative Care

Cherny, N. I. "Update in the Management of Cancer Pain." In *Principles and Practice of Supportive Oncology* edited by A. M. Berger, R. K. Portenoy, and D. E. Weissman. New York: Lipincott Williams & Wilkins Healthcare 1 (1999): 1–16.

Jadad, A. R. and G. P. Browman. "The WHO Analgesic Ladder for Cancer Pain Management: Stepping up the Quality of Its Evaluation." *Journal of the American Medical Association* 274 (1995): 1870–1873.

O'Neill, B. and M. Fallon. "ABC of Palliative Care: Principles of Palliative Care and Pain Control." *British Medical Journal* 315 (1997): 801–804.

Redefining Addiction in Palliative Settings

Bruera, E. and C. Sweeney. "Methadone Use in Cancer Patients with Pain: A Review." *Journal of Palliative Medicine* 5 (2002): 127–138.

Passik, S. D., K. L. Kirsh, and R. K. Portenoy. "Understanding Aberrant Drug-Taking Behavior: Addiction Redefined for Palliative Care and Pain Management Settings." In *Principles and Practice of Supportive Oncology* edited by A. M. Berger, R. K. Portenoy, and D. E. Weissman. New York: Lipincott Williams & Wilkins Healthcare 2 (1999): 1–12.

Pain Management in the Elderly

M. D. Anderson Cancer Center Pain Research Group. " Undertreatment of Cancer Pain in Elderly Patients." *Journal of the American Medical Association* 279 (1998): 1914–1915.

Weissman, E. D., J. Griffie, S. Muchka, and S. Matson. "Improving Pain Management in Long-term Care Facilities." *Journal of Palliative Care* 4 (2001): 567–573.

Palliation of Non-End-of-Life Pain Syndromes

Baumrucker, S. J. "Post-Thoracotomy Pain Syndrome: An Opportunity for Palliative Care." *American Journal of Hospice and Palliative Care* 19 (2002): 83–86.

1.12 Opioid Side Effects

Key Points

1. Treatment of pain with opioids includes monitoring for multiple side effects. Opioid side effects include sedation, constipation, nausea/vomiting, delirium, urinary retention, multifocal myoclonus, respiratory depression, withdrawal/physical dependence, acetaminophen or aspirin overdose, cost and diversion of medications. Have medications available to manage side effects.

2. As a general rule, begin with short-acting opioids and switch back to them with the development of dehydration or renal/hepatic failure or during the active dying phase.
   Review other medications when starting opioid. Pay special attention to dosing when oral route no longer possible.

3. The benefit of pain relief may outweigh the burden of side effects that cannot be completely controlled.

4. Constipation, which is not self-limiting, is a side effect of opioids.
   Constipation is easier to prevent than to treat. Counter constipation with a large-bowel stimulant such as Biscodyl or Senna. Goal is a bowel movement at least QOD.

5. Delirium is a side effect of opioids.
   Counter delirium by considering other causes and rotation of opioid to short-acting form. The physician may need to treat through the delirium if the option is poorly controlled pain.

6. Respiratory depression is a rare side effect of opioids, usually occurring only in opioid-naive patients in whom tolerance develops quickly.
   Begin with short-acting opioids and small doses. Sedation usually precedes respiratory depression.

7. Cost/access barriers to procuring opioids can lead to pseudo-addictive behaviors.
   Patients may have difficulty affording opioids; generic drugs are usually less expensive. Patients may have difficulty accessing opioids because of the requirement for a written refill, Medicaid/insurance limits on maximum doses, failure of pharmacies to carry certain medications, and time limits on frequency of refills that may preclude a prescribed dose escalation.

Opioid Side Effects

The Palliative Response

Types of Opioids

- Tylenol/Codeine (Tylenol #3™)
- Tylenol/Hydrocodone (Lortab™)
- Tylenol/Oxycodone (Vicodin™, Percocet™)
- Aspirin/Oxycodone (Percodan™)
- Propoxyphene (Darvon™, Darvocet™)
- Methadone (Dolophine™)
- Morphine (MS Contin™, Oromorp™, Roxicet™, Roxinol™)
- Hydromorphone (Dilaudid™)
- Fentanyl (Duragesic™)

Opioid Routes and Forms

- Oral
- Sublingual
- Subcutaneous
- Rectal
- Topical
- Intramuscular
- Intravenous
- Intraspinal
- Liquid
- Concentrate
- Immediate release
- Sustained release
- Suppository
- Injection
- Infusion
- PCA (patient-controlled)

Factors That May Affect Opioid Dosing

- Renal failure
- Hepatic failure
- Advanced age
- History of substance abuse
- Concomitant medications
- Dehydration
- Route
- Last hours of life

Side Effects to Monitor

- Sedation
- Constipation
- Nausea/vomiting
- Delirium
- Urinary retention
- Myoclonus, multifocal
- Respiratory depression
- Withdrawal/physical dependence
- Tylenol overdose
- Aspirin overdose
- Cost
- Diversion of medications

General Principles of Side-Effect Management

- Anticipate side effects
  Have medications available to manage
- Warn/counsel patients about side effects
  Many side effects are self-limiting
  Call-back may be helpful at 24–48 hours to advise patients about management of opioids
  Counsel against exceeding 4 grams Tylenol/24 hours (Many patients are not aware that they should not use Tylenol and combination opioids together)

General Principles of Opioid Dosing

- Initiating opioids
  Review medications when starting opioid
  As general rule, begin with short-acting opioids and convert to sustained-release after a dose finding
- Switch back to short-acting opioids when:
  Dehydration develops
  Renal or hepatic failure develops
  Patient is in the actively dying phase
- Special attention to dosing when oral route no longer possible

Opioids
Burden versus Benefit

- Some side effects will develop during treatment of pain with opioids
- Patient and healthcare provider should discuss ways to minimize side effects
- However, the benefit of pain relief may outweigh the burden of the side effects if they cannot be completely controlled

Opioid Side Effect: Sedation

- Many patients who have been sleep-deprived by poorly controlled pain, sleep more than usual in the first few days after starting an opioid

- Sedation is usually self-limiting

Countering Sedation

- Discontinue or reduce other sedating medications when feasible
- Consider switching to shorter-acting opioids if pharmacological accumulation is of concern
- Reduce dose
- Consider methylphenidate 2.5–5mg 2 or 3 times during day
- Discuss patient's preference for sedation versus level of pain control

Opioid Side Effect: Constipation

- Not a self-limiting side effect
- Goal: Prevent versus treat
  Start a laxative when start an opioid
  Consider discontinuing or altering other medications that may cause constipation
- Countering constipation
  Use a large-bowel stimulant as a laxative (e.g., biscodyl or senna)
  Goal is a bowel movement at least QOD

Opioid Side Effect: Nausea/Vomiting

- Usually self-limiting

- Action of opioids
  Affect chemoreceptor trigger zone
  Delay gastric emptying

Countering Nausea/ Vomiting

- Consider premedicating
  Use caution about sedating effects of combination treatment
- Consider metochlopromide or haloperidol
- For persistent nausea/vomiting, rotate to alternative route or equivalent dose of another opioid

Persistent Nausea/ Vomiting
Differential Diagnosis

- Other medications
- Constipation
- Obstruction
- Progression of the illness

Opioid Side Effect:
Urinary Retention

- High-risk patients – monitor for retention
  History of retention
  BPH in elderly
  Patients on medications (e.g., anticholinergics) that may contribute to urinary retention
- Countering urinary retention
  Foley catheter
  Consider stopping other medications
  Treat infection
  Treat with Terazosin (Hytrin)

Opioid Side Effect:
Multifocal Myoclonus

- Countering Multifocal Myoclonus
  Opioid rotation
  Reduce dose if pain will allow
  Try to maintain hydration
  Stop long-acting and continuous opioids
  Benzodiazepines
- Differential diagnosis
  Consider that renal or hepatic dysfunction may be developing

Opioid Side Effect:
Delirium

- Consider and treat other causes for delirium
- Treat delirium with haloperidol
- Rotate opioid and switch to short-acting form
- Fentanyl
  Has many advantages but...
  May be problematic because of accumulation in lipid-rich areas like the brain
- May need to treat through the delirium if the option is poorly controlled pain

Opioid Side Effect:
Respiratory Depression

- Presentation
  Usually opioid-naive patients
  Tolerance develops quickly
- Prevention
  Begin with short-acting opioids, small doses
- Forewarning
  Sedation usually precedes respiratory depression

Opioid Side Effect:
Respiratory Depression

High-Risk Patients

- Treated for acute pain now resolved
- Debilitation
- Neurological impairment
- Respiratory impairment
- New onset of renal or hepatic insufficiency

Respiratory Depression
Treatment

- Prevent by holding doses for sedation if pain control is adequate
- Opioid rotation may be helpful (less helpful than for other side effects)
- Naloxone
  Use with caution—can cause acute withdrawal and pain crisis

  10:1 dilution with careful titration

Respiratory Depression
Burden versus Benefit

- Some degree of sedation may be acceptable to patient/family in cases where pain is difficult to control

Opioid Side Effect:
Withdrawal/Dependence

- Withdrawal effects in patients treated with opioids for chronic pain
- Withdrawal may precipitate
  Pain crisis

  Physical withdrawal
- Examples of withholding
  Complication of disease that prevents oral dosing

  Hospital admission

Opioid Side Effect:
Tylenol/Aspirin Overdose

- Overdose from combination opioids
  Patient may take too much acetaminophen secondary to ineffective pain treatment so that they escalate combination opioid unaware of danger
- Overdose from Tylenol/Aspirin
  Patient may add these drugs to a combination out of ignorance about potential results

Opioid Side Effect:
Cost/Access Barrier

- Cost barriers
- Access barriers
  Opioids require written refill

  Medicaid/insurance limits on maximum doses

  Many pharmacies do not carry certain medications

  Time limits on frequency of refills (may affect patient who needed a dose escalation during the previous month)
- Barriers can lead to pseudo-addictive behaviors

Opioid Side Effects

Selected Readings

Patient's Experience of Pain

Weiss, S. C., L. L. Emanuel, D. L. Fairclough, and E. J. Emanuel. "Understanding the Experience of Pain in Terminally Ill Patients." *The Lancet* 357 (2001): 1311–1315.

Classification of Cancer Pain

Caraceni, A. and S. M. Weinstein. "Classification of Cancer Pain Syndromes." *Oncology* 15 (2001): 1627–1639.

Management of Pain in Palliative Care

Cherny, N. I. "Update in the Management of Cancer Pain." In *Principles and Practice of Supportive Oncology* edited by A. M. Berger, R. K. Portenoy, and D. E. Weissman. New York: Lipincott Williams & Wilkins Healthcare, 1 (1999): 1–16.

Jadad, A. R. and G. P. Browman. "The WHO Analgesic Ladder for Cancer Pain Management: Stepping up the Quality of Its Evaluation." *Journal of the American Medical Association* 274 (1995): 1870–1873.

O'Neill, B. and M. Fallon. "ABC of Palliative Care: Principles of Palliative Care and Pain Control." *British Medical Journal* 315 (1997): 801–804.

Redefining Addiction in Palliative Settings

Bruera, E. and C. Sweeney. "Methadone Use in Cancer Patients with Pain: A Review." *Journal of Palliative Medicine* 5 (2002): 127–138.

Passik, S. D., K. L. Kirsh, and R. K. Portenoy. "Understanding Aberrant Drug-Taking Behavior: Addiction Redefined for Palliative Care and Pain Management Settings." In *Principles and Practice of Supportive Oncology* edited by A. M. Berger, R. K. Portenoy, and D. E. Weissman. New York: Lipincott Williams & Wilkins Healthcare, 2 (1999): 1–12.

Pain Management in the Elderly

M. D. Anderson Cancer Center Pain Research Group. "Undertreatment of Cancer Pain in Elderly Patients." *Journal of the American Medical Association* 279 (1998): 1914–1915.

Weissman, E. D., J. Griffie, S. Muchka, and S. Matson. "Improving Pain Management in Long-term Care Facilities." *Journal of Palliative Care* 4 (2001): 567–573.

Palliation of Non-End-of-Life Pain Syndromes

Baumrucker, S. J. "Post-Thoracotomy Pain Syndrome: An Opportunity for Palliative Care." *American Journal of Hospice and Palliative Care* 19 (2002): 83–86.

1.13 Pressure Ulcers

Key Points

1. Pressure ulcers cause pain for patients and distress for family, and they negatively impact both quality and quantity of life.

2. Prevention is the key for effectively managing pressure ulcers.
   Evaluate all patients frequently and follow an active plan for both prevention and treatment. Consult with a skin-care nurse for management advice.

3. Stage 1 pressure ulcers present as changes in intact skin and require prompt attention to prevent skin breakdown and ulcer development.
   Visual evidence is discoloration, redness, and bogginess of intact skin. Sensory evidence is pain, warmth, and itchiness.

4. Stage 2 pressure ulcers present as epidermal loss forming shallow crater, abrasion, or blister. Stage 2 pressure ulcers can quickly progress to Stage 3.
   With treatment and removal of pressure, Stage 2 ulcer may heal over a 7–10 day period.

5. Stage 3 pressure ulcers present as full-thickness tissue loss to facia with a deep crater. Stage 3 pressure ulcers require debridement and special dressing. Healing from viable skin on edges of the wound can take weeks to months and may never occur in severely debilitated patients at Life's End.

6. Stage 4 pressure ulcers present as full-thickness loss of skin with visible bone, muscle, or tendons. Stage 4 pressure ulcers impact negatively on survival.
   Stage 4 ulcers may be associated with osteomyelitis and undermining of skin and sinus tracts.

7. Prevention is the key to managing pressure ulcers at Life's End.
   Screen all patients for presence of ulcers. Scan all skin surfaces with special attention to high-risk sites: sacrum, heels, ankles, hips, knees, elbows, and ears. Record stage of ulcers, risk of progression, and plan of care.
   Control physical symptoms to help keep patient mobile and to reduce risk of ulcer development.

Pressure Ulcers

The Palliative Response

Impact

Incidence
- High risk for all patients at Life's End

Suffering
- Pain for patients
- Distress for family
- Negative impact on quality and quantity of life

Pressure Ulcers: The Palliative Response

Prevention is the key to care for pressure ulcers at Life's End.

Intervention

- Evaluate all palliative patients frequently
- Prevent and treat with active plans
- Consult skin-care nurse for management advice

Pressure Ulcers Stage 1

Evaluation
- Visual evidence
  Discoloration, redness, bogginess of intact skin
- Sensory evidence
  Pain, warmth, itchiness

Treatment
- Address promptly in effort to prevent breakdown and development of ulcer

---

Pressure Ulcers Stage 2

Evaluation
- Skin no longer intact
- Epidermal loss forms shallow crater, abrasion, or blister

Prognosis with Treatment
- Can progress to Stage 3 in 24–48 hours
- May heal over 7–10 days with treatment and removal of pressure

Pressure Ulcers
Stage 3

Evaluation

- Deep crater—full-thickness tissue loss to fascia

Treatment and Prognosis

- Debridement and special dressing for comfort and to prevent progression
- Healing from viable skin on edges of wound can take weeks to months
- Ulcers may never heal in severely debilitated patients at Life's End

Pressure Ulcers
Stage 4

Evaluation

- Visible bone, muscle, and/or tendons—full-thickness loss of skin
- May be associated with osteomyelitis and undermining of skin and sinus tracts

Prognosis

- Often cause tremendous suffering

Pressure Ulcers
Considerations

Evaluation

- Determination of staging may require debridement if necrotic tissue (e.g., eschar) present

Treatment

- Selected patients may benefit from surgical treatment
- Most palliative care patients are not candidates for flaps or other plastic surgery procedures

Screen
for Pressure Ulcers

Screen all skin surface at Life's End

High-risk sites:
- Sacrum
- Heels
- Ankles
- Hips
- Knees
- Elbows
- Ears

Record Pressure Ulcers

- Stage of ulcer
- Risk of progression
- Plan of care

Control Symptoms

Control of physical symptoms helps keep patient mobile and reduces risk of ulcer development.

Risk Factors: Mobility and Activity

Lower risk
- Patients who are up and out of bed

Higher risk
- Bedridden patients
- Patients whose mobility in bed is restricted (restraints, compression devises on legs, oxygen)
- Patients who tend to move less (secondary to pain or other poorly controlled symptoms)

Risk Factors: Moisture from Incontinence

Intervention for prevention
- Change diapers and pad as needed
- Clean linens
- Cleanse skin
- Apply moisture barrier ointments
- Use bladder catheter if necessary—avoid if possible

Risk Factors: Sensory Impairment

- Decreased level of consciousness or sensory impairment due to neuropathy or cord injury

- Prevents normal response of sensing pressure and changing position to relieve pressure and protect skin integrity

Risk Factors: Declining Nutrition

Palliative response
- Assess barriers to adequate oral intake
- Treat anorexia
- Avoid invasive nutritional support
  Does not seem to improve outcome
  Does not seem to prevent ulcers
  May complicate care with reduced mobility
  May increase moisture from diarrhea/ urinary output

Risk Factors: Skin Shear

Evaluation
- Fragile skin damaged by friction and tearing with movement

Treatment
- Use draw sheet and other devises to protect skin with movement
- Employ protective devices (padding, wedges, heel protectors)

Pressure Ulcers: The Palliative Response

Prevention is the key.

Control physical symptoms to help keep patient mobile and reduce risk of ulcer development at Life's End.

Pressure Ulcers

Selected Readings

Hess, C. T. "Fundamental Strategies for Skin Care: A Comprehensive Understanding of Skin and Topical Products Is Essential in Maintaining a Patient's Skin Integrity." Ostomy/Wound Management 43 (1997): 3–41.

Walker, P. W. "Update on Pressure Ulcers." In Principles and Practice of Supportive Oncology edited by A. M. Berger, R. K. Portenoy, and D. E. Weissman. New York: Lipincott Williams & Wilkins Healthcare 3 (2000): 1–11.

1.14 Intentional Sedation

Key Points

1. The intended result of intentional sedation, also called sedation at Life's End and terminal sedation, is to achieve comfort in a decreased level of consciousness when a patient at Life's End suffers from unrelieved and unbearable symptoms despite treatment.

   The physician will not need to consider intentional sedation frequently if symptoms are well controlled. More than 95% of patients with pain can achieve adequate relief with standard therapies.

2. Weigh burden and benefits of intentional sedation, including perceptions of patient and family regarding burden of suffering; consider all reasonable alternatives for symptom relief; seek consultation of multidisciplinary team; and scrupulously document considerations.

3. Serious moral implications extend to withholding as well as administering, sedation in patients with unrelieved suffering at Life's End.

   Clarity on cause of death aids consideration. The underlying illness, not any treatment provided by the medical team, causes the patient's death.

4. Intentional sedation involves the principle of double effect (all actions may have both positive and negative effects and a specific action is ethical if the intent is for patient's benefit) and follows the ethical principles of autonomy, beneficence, and non-maleficence.

   The physician provides medical care consistent with the Goals of Care of the patient and family and with the best and most appropriate treatment for a patient whose suffering is unrelievable and unbearable. The physician avoids harmful treatments, assures that DNAR orders are written, and that orders for analgesic medicines do not expire.

5. Intentional sedation, a palliative treatment of last resort to relieve suffering, differs ethically and in practice from physician-assisted suicide (PAS) and euthanasia.

   In PAS, legal only in Oregon, the intention of both physician and patient is death rather than the relief of unbearable symptoms. In fact, most patients who avail themselves of PAS do so to maintain a sense of control over their dying and in anticipation of future symptoms. In euthanasia, which is legally considered murder and never considered ethical, the physician's intention is the patient's death rather than the relief of unbearable symptoms.

Intentional Sedation

The Palliative Response

Mr. Johnson's Case

Diagnosis and Status of Disease
- Widely metastatic non-small-cell lung cancer
- No longer responsive to treatment

Symptoms
- Severe pain from spread of tumor to bone
- Dyspnea due to lung damage from both the tumor and past treatment

Prognosis
- Grave: Life expectancy probably hours to days
- Medical team, patient, and family are all aware

Mr. Johnson's Course of Palliation

- Admission to palliative-care unit
- Symptom-control efforts with all available and appropriate treatments
- Symptoms unrelieved and, by Mr. Johnson's description, unbearable
- Suffering relieved only when sedated with medication that the team is trying to titrate to control the pain and delirium

---

Mr. Johnson's Status with Palliation

- Not eating or drinking much fluid
- Bed confined
- Continued on medication combination

  Opioid

  Benzodiazepine

  Neuroleptic
- Pain and dyspnea seem to be relieved; he seems to be sleeping
- Mr. Johnson dies 3 days later

Intentional Sedation: Definition

Process and intention
- Administer medication at Life's End to induce sedation, sleep-like state, decreased consciousness

Indication
- Unrelieved/unbearable suffering from pain, dyspnea, delirium, etc. despite efforts
- Usually considered only when prognosis is hours to days or days to a few weeks

Other names
- Terminal sedation, sedation at Life's End

Role of Good Pain Control

- The physician will not need to consider Intentional Sedation frequently if symptoms are well controlled

- Greater than 95% of patients with pain can achieve adequate pain relief with standard therapies

---

Moral Considerations

- Consider moral implications

- Consider all reasonable avenues to relieve symptoms causing suffering

- Consider burden/risk of Intentional Sedation

  Balance with potential benefits

  Consider perceptions of patient/ family regarding the burden of suffering

Seeking Consultation

- Access expertise of the multi-disciplinary palliative care team

- Pastoral care often plays an important role in consideration of Intentional Sedation

  Care for patient, family, clinical team as unit

- Ethics committee

  Consult may be helpful but not required in considering Intentional Sedation

Moral Implications
Withholding Sedation

Serious moral implications of withholding, as well as administering, sedation in patients with unrelieved suffering at Life's End

- Clarity on cause of death may help clarify the consideration
- The underlying illness, not the treatment, causes the patient's death

The Principle of Double Effect

- Reality of double effect

  All actions may have both positive and negative effects

- Determination of ethicalness

  A specific action is ethical if the intent of that action is for the patient's benefit even though a negative effect may occur

Purpose
Sedation versus PAS

- Purpose of intentional sedation

  To alleviate unrelieved, unbearable suffering with medication administered by physician

- Purpose of physician-assisted suicide

  To assure that the patient will die as a result of medication provided by physician

Ethical Consideration
Autonomy

- Consult and inform

  Physician should consult and inform patient—or surrogate if patient has lost capacity—about treatment options

- Honor preferences

  Experience of suffering and ability to bear suffering are highly subjective and individual

  Some patients and families choose to accept increased sedation in the face of unrelieved suffering

Ethical Consideration
Beneficence

Intention of medical provider
- To provide medical care consistent with the Goals of Care of patient and family

- To provide the best and most appropriate treatment for a patient whose suffering is unrelieved and unbearable at Life's End

Ethical Consideration
Non-Maleficence

Intention of medical provider
- To avoid harmful treatment for patients
- Examples

  Avoid harmful interventions

  Assure that Do Not Attempt to Resuscitate orders are written

  Assure that orders for analgesic medicines do not expire

Intentional Sedation Is <u>Not</u> Physician-Assisted Suicide

- Level of acceptance of PAS

  A legal option only in Oregon
- Prevalence of PAS

  Most patients avail themselves of PAS to maintain a sense of control over their dying

  Reasons for PAS are usually not primarily the current symptoms but the anticipation of future symptoms

Intentional Sedation Is <u>Not</u> Physician-Assisted Suicide

- Timing of PAS

  More likely considered with grave prognosis

  More likely weeks to even months before anticipated death
- Intention of PAS

  Death versus relief of unbearable symptoms

Intentional Sedation Is <u>Not</u> Euthanasia

- Process and intention of euthanasia

  Physician administers medication

  Physician's intent is that patient will die

- Ethics of euthanasia

  Euthanasia is never considered ethical

  Euthanasia is legally considered murder

Intentional Sedation
The Palliative Response

- Palliative treatment to relieve suffering

  Treatment of last resort

  Openly discuss

  Scrupulously document

- Contrast with PAS and euthanasia

  Differs ethically

  Differs in practice

Selected Readings

Definition and Review of Terminal Sedation in Palliative Medicine

Cowan, J. D. and D. Walsh. "Terminal Sedation in Palliative Medicine—Definition and Review of the Literature." Comment in *Supportive Care Cancer* 9 (2001): 401–402, 403–407.

Intentional Sedation as Response to Intractable Terminal Suffering

Chater, S., R. Viola, J. Paterson, and V. Jarvis. "Sedation for Intractable Distress in the Dying: A Survey of Experts." *Palliative Medicine* 12 (1998): 255–269.

Cherny, N. I. "The Use of Sedation in the Management of Refractory Pain." In *Principles and Practice of Supportive Oncology* edited by A. M. Berger, R. K. Portenoy, and D. E. Weissman. New York: Lipincott Williams & Wilkins Healthcare, 3 (2000): 1–11.

Quill, T. E. and I. R. Byock. "Responding to Intractable Terminal Suffering: the Role of Terminal Sedation and Voluntary Refusal of Food and Fluids." *Annals of Internal Medicine* 132 (2000): 408–414.

Terminal Sedation for Existential Distress

Morita, T., J. Tsunoda, S. Inoue, and S. Chihara. "Terminal Sedation for Existential Distress." Comment in *American Journal of Hospice and Palliative Care* 17 (2000): 148–149, 189–195.

Sedation in the Imminently Dying Patient

Wein, S. "Sedation in the Imminently Dying Patient." *Oncology* 14 (2000): 585–590.

What's in a Name?

Jackson, W. C. "Palliative Sedation vs. Terminal Sedation: What's in a Name?" *American Journal of Hospice and Palliative Care* 19 (2002): 81–82.

1.15 Last Hours of Life (I and II)

Key Points

1. The Goals of Care in the last hours of life are comfort, support, and protection from iatrogenic harm.

2. Continuing to "do everything" for the patient can contribute to physical, emotional, social, and spiritual/existential suffering. Common interventions at Life's End include:
   - IV fluids and central lines; blood work, arterial blood gas and imaging studies
   - Nasogastric tubes, peg tubes, and TPN; bladder catheters and rectal tubes
   - Oxygen therapy mask, non-rebreather, and BiPAP
   - Intubation, suctioning, nasal trumpet, nebulizations, oxygen saturation monitoring, arterial line, and telemetry
   - CPR and attempted resuscitation; restraints
   - Separation from family and loved ones

3. DNAR (Do Not Attempt Resuscitation) or AND (Allow Natural Death) are preferable to DNR (Do Not Resuscitate) as orders.
   DNR suggests that medical personnel can successfully resuscitate at Life's End but choose not to do so. Resuscitation is not an effective treatment in End-of-Life Care.

4. Assist the family by advising when to call other family members in, writing orders to facilitate visiting or staying, and educating them about physical markers of life's final days.
   Arrange visits for military relatives by contacting the Red Cross and for incarcerated relatives by contacting prison wardens. Give families the pamphlet *Gone from My Sight* as a guide to the last days of life.

Last Hours of Life (I)

The Palliative Response

Mr. Edward Johnson Is Dying

- 75-year-old widower

- Diagnosed with stage IV non-small-cell lung cancer six months ago. Now has progressive disease despite chemotherapy and radiation therapy.

- Brought to the ER
  Uncontrolled pain
  Has not been getting out of bed

Physical Exam
of Mr. Johnson

- Thin male with temporal wasting
- Blue tinged lips and nail
- BP 80/40 P140 RR30 T100.2
- 4x4cm lymph node in R supraclavicular space
- Coarse breath sounds in all lung fields and dullness R base
- Liver 10cm below the R rib margin
- Tender 3+ edema to the knees

Assessment
of Mr. Johnson

- Mr. Johnson is terminally ill with progressive lung cancer, an illness man cannot cure

- Mr. Johnson is not responding to disease-modifying treatments

Goals of Care
for Mr. Johnson

- Comfort

- Support

- Protection from iatrogenic harm

Reflection
Suffering Paradigm

Make a list of symptoms or problems that you anticipate might cause suffering for Mr. Johnson and his family during this phase of his illness.

Reflection
Physical Suffering

What *Physical Suffering* do you anticipate during this phase of Mr. Johnson's illness?

Reflection
Emotional Suffering

What *Emotional Suffering* do you anticipate during this phase of Mr. Johnson's illness?

Reflection
Social Suffering

What *Social Suffering* do you anticipate during this phase of Mr. Johnson's illness?

Reflection
Spiritual/Existential Suffering

What *Spiritual/Existential* Suffering do you anticipate during this phase of Mr. Johnson's illness?

"Do Everything"

- Your team has been called to the ER to admit Mr. Johnson

- ER physician informs you that the family has already left

  Before they left, she asked them if they wanted the doctors to "do everything"

  They said "Yes"

- She has called for a bed in the ICU

ICU Interventions

- Reflect on the kinds of treatments and interventions that might be anticipated in the ICU when you "do everything"

- List anticipated interventions

Impact of Interventions

What impact do you anticipate that these interventions will have on Mr. Johnson's suffering at Life's End?

- Physical
- Emotional
- Social
- Spiritual/Existential

Sources of Suffering
at Life's End

Physical
- Pain
- Dyspnea
- Anorexia
- Nausea/Vomiting
- Constipation
- Asthenia
- Skin breakdown
- Dysphagia
- Problems with secretions
- Incontinence

Sources of Suffering
at Life's End

Emotional
- Delirium
- Depression
- Anxiety

Social
- Lack of financial resource
- Inadequate housing
- Lack of full-time caregiver

Spiritual/Existential
- Spiritual anguish
- Loss of meaning

Common Interventions
at Life's End

- IV fluids and central lines
- Blood work, arterial blood gas, imaging studies
- Nasogastric tubes, peg tubes, TPN
- Bladder catheters and rectal tubes
- Oxygen therapy mask, non-rebreather, BiPAP

Common Interventions
at Life's End

- Intubation, suctioning, nasal trumpet, nebulizations, oxygen saturation monitoring, arterial line, telemetry
- CPR and attempted resuscitation
- Restraints
- Separation from family/loved ones

To be continued in

Last Hours of Life (II)

Last Hours of Life (II)

Annotated Orders for Comfort Care

Admission

- Admit and initiate Comfort Care Order Set or
- Transfer and initiate Comfort Care Order Set or
- Initiate Comfort Care Order Set
- Diagnosis: Metastatic Lung Cancer/Pain Crisis
- Condition: Grave
- Status: Do Not Attempt Resuscitation (DNAR)
- Orders: Focus on <u>what you can do</u> that may be helpful

Do Not Attempt Resuscitation

Resuscitation is not an effective treatment at Life's End

- DNAR terminology preferable to DNR
- DNR (Do Not Resuscitate) suggests that one can successfully resuscitate at Life's End but chooses not to do so

Diet

- Order a diet
  Patient may improve and desire the taste of food
- Full liquid instead of clear liquid
  More palatable
  Easier to swallow, less likely to cause aspiration
  Can advance if tolerated
- May have food brought in by family
- Allow patient to sit up for meals; assist to eat
  Use dietary and nursing care text orders in CCOS to select most appropriate orders

Activity

- Allow patient to sit in chair if desired

- Allow patient to use bedside commode if safe

- Allow family to stay in room with patient
  Use nursing care text orders to select theses or other appropriate orders for patient and family comfort.

  Avoid orders for strict bed rest.

Vital Signs

- Minimum frequency allowed by policy (usually not more than once a shift)
- Limit notification orders to those necessary
  Frequent monitoring can alarm patient and family
  Numbers can distract staff/family from patient
  The goal at Life's End is symptom control, not getting a number
  Use the notification orders in CCOS to review options such as
  Call MD if pain not controlled or family needs to speak to physician

IV Considerations

- Starting is often difficult and painful
- Often has no benefit for patient
- Many patients have fluid overload, edema, and pulmonary congestion
- Many patients have limited movement in bed and are restrained to protect the IV
- Oral hydration is a reasonable compromise. If IV fluids are used, suggest a limited time trial, such as a 1000–1500cc D5½ NS over 6 hours.
- Presence of edema indicates that patient is not dehydrated

Subcutaneous (SQ) Line

- Small IV needle inserted directly under the skin, often on the abdomen or thigh
- Small volumes of many medicines can be injected when the oral route is not available
- Avoids burden of finding and maintaining IV access

Hypodermoclysis

- Technique for giving ½NS at 30–45 cc/hour continuous for rehydration, using the SQ route when an IV route may be burdensome
  Use nursing care text and IV order options in CCOS to select patient

Dyspnea

- Oxygen 2–4l nasal prong

- Usually do not use mask

- Usually do monitor oxygen saturation
  Use respiratory care options in CCOS to select patient-specific orders

Persistent Dyspnea

- Blow air on face with bedside fan
- Morphine for dyspnea such as MS 2–4 mg IV/SQ q2 hours respiratory rate > 20/minutes
- Turning, repositioning, sitting up
- Nebs may help
  But can lead to tachycardia and anxiety from the beta agonist
- Avoid face mask
  *Most patients will not tolerate
  Interferes with communication
  Increases use of restraints
  Use nursing care text and opioid order options in CCOS to select patient-specific orders*

Hygiene

- Avoid Foley catheter if possible
  *Try diapers and cleansing instead
  Delirious patient may pull on bladder catheter
  May be helpful for hygiene (e.g., obesity) but same thing may be accomplished with diapers. Catheters may be more appropriate if patient is in significant pain with movement (e.g., multiple bone lesions or fractured hip)*
- Check all patients for impaction
  Suppository may be helpful
- Consider evaluation by skin-care nurse
  Use nursing care text and medication order options in CCOS to select patient-specific orders

Pain and Dyspnea

- Opioids usually most effective
- Calculate morphine equivalents used in recent past; adjust as needed
- Usually will want to stop sustained-release medicines and use immediate-release medications

Morphine concentrate 20mg/ml

- Start with MS 5mg–20 mg q2 sub-lingual hours (*Offer/Patient May Refuse*)
- Or Morphine Sulfate SQ/IV q2 hours (1/3 the oral dose) (*Offer/Patient May Refuse*)
- Or Morphine Sulfate continuous infusion 1–3 mg/hour (titrate to patient's comfort)
  Use opioid medication order options in CCOS to select patient-specific orders

Pain, Dyspnea, Anorexia, Asthenia, and Depression

Dexamethasone

- Can have multiple beneficial effects
- Most complications are long-term (over a year or more) and not a concern in patients at Life's End
- Less mineral-corticoid effect than Prednisone
- Does not have to be given in multiple doses

Dexamethasone 4mg PO/SQ/IV BID at breakfast and lunch

Use Dexamethasone medication order options in CCOS to select patient-specific orders

Nausea and Delirium

Haloperidol

- Excellent antiemitic
- Chemically related to chlorpromazine but less sedating
- Helpful with delirium common at Life's End
  a. Haloperidol 2mg PO or 1mg SQ/IV q2 hours, x 3 doses or until settled, then q6–8 hours PRN
  b. Patient > 65 years: Haloperidol 1mg PO or 0.5 mg SQ/IV q2 hours, x 3 doses or until settled, then q6–8 hours PRN
- Nausea usually requires less frequent doses

Use Haloperidol medication order options in CCOS to select patient-specific orders

Anxiety and Seizures

Lorazepam

- May be helpful with anxiety
- Exercise care as delirium can sometimes be mistaken for anxiety; benzodiazepines may make delirium worse
- Effective against seizures only as IV or SQ not PO

a. Lorazepam 1mg PO or SQ q6–8 hours PRN

b. Patients > 65 years old Lorazepam 0.5–1mg PO or SQ q6–8 hours PRN

Use Lorazepam medication order options in CCOS to select patient-specific orders

Death Rattle

- Turn and reposition to the side
- Stop IV fluids or tube feeding
- Scopolamine patch topical behind ear q3 days
- Atropine eye drops 2–3gtts in mouth q4 hours or until patch effective
- Avoid deep suctioning but Yonkers might help with mouth care
- Sponge sticks with soda wash to cleanse mouth every 2–4 hours. Family can be engaged to help.

Use secretion medication order options in CCOS to select patient-specific orders

Tips for Comfort and Safety

Comforting Measures

- Reposition
- Massage
- Quietly sit with and speak to patient
- Soft music

Minimize Discomfort

- Avoid sensory overload (e.g., TV)
- Use bed-minder in lieu of restraints to alarm if patient gets up

Assisting Family

- Advise family about alerting other loved ones about the gravity of patient's status
- Facilitate family presence
  Order permission for family to visit or stay
  Arrange visits for military (contact Red Cross) and incarcerated relatives (contact warden)
- Consult Pastoral Care and Social Work
- Provide family with pamphlet on dying process

Use consult order options in CCOS to select patient-specific orders

Last Hours of Life

Selected Readings

Overview of Symptom Management in the Last Hours of Life

Adam, J. "ABC of Palliative Care: The Last 48 Hours." *British Medical Journal* 315 (1997): 1600–1603.

Quality Control of Care in Last Hours of Life

Ellershaw, J., C. Smith, S. Overill, S. E. Walker, and J. Aldridge. "Care of the Dying: Setting Standards for Symptom Control in the Last 48 Hours of Life." *Journal of Pain and Symptom Management* 21 (2001): 12–17.

Ferris, F. D., C. F. von Gunten, and L. L. Emanuel. "Ensuring Competency in End-of-Life Care: Controlling Symptoms." *BMC Palliattive Care* 1 (2002): 5.

Managing Specific Symptoms in the Last Hours of Life

Perkin, R. M. and D. B. Resnik. "The Agony of Agonal Respiration: Is the Last Gasp Necessary?" *Journal of Medical Ethics* 28 (2002): 164–169.

Stirling, L. C., A. Kurowska, and A. Tookman. "The Use of Phenobarbital in the Management of Agitation and Seizures at the End of Life." *Journal of Pain and Symptom Management* 17 (1999): 363–368. Comment in 19 (2000): 80–81.

Ventafridda, V., C. Ripamonti, F. De Conno, M. Tamburini, and B. R. Cassileth. "Symptom Prevalence and Control During Cancer Patients' Last Days of Life." *Journal of Palliative Care* 6 (1990): 7–11. Comment in 7 (1991): 50–51.

Implications for End-of-Life Decision Making

Sykes, N. and A. Thorns. "Sedative Use in the Last Week of Life and the Implications for End-of-Life Decision Making." *Archives of Internal Medicine* 163 (2003): 341–344.

Managing Terminal Symptoms in Non-Hospital Settings

Hall, P., D. Schroder, and L. Weaver. "The Last 48 Hours of Life in Long-term Care: A Focused Chart Audit." *Journal of the American Geriatrics Society* 50 (2002): 501–506.

LeGrand, S. B., P. Tropiano, J. D. Marx, M. P. Davis, and D. Walsh. "Dying at Home: Emergency Medications for Terminal Symptoms." *American Journal of Hospice and Palliative Care* 18 (2001): 421–423.

Estimating Number of Dying Patients in Hospital

Billings, J. A., M. Gardner, and A. T. Putnam. "A One-Day, Hospital-Wide Survey of Dying Inpatients." *Journal of Palliative Medicine* 5 (2002): 363–374.

1.16   Debility

Key Points

1. Debility is a condition of declining functional status with limited prognosis and sometimes multiple diagnoses in the absence of any one terminal illness.

   While no one knows how long anyone will live, there are certain signs that health is very poor and declining and that time could be limited.

2. To predict life expectancy as accurately as possible, ask, "Would I be surprised if this patient died in the next six months?" Language is very important in discussing prognosis and hospice referral.

   "Because of the severity of your illness, you and your family are eligible for the assistance of hospice at home" is preferable to "You have a prognosis of less than six months. Therefore, I am referring you to hospice."

3. Markers for poor prognosis include disease progression, multiple ER and/or hospital admissions, increased dependence, or need for home-care services.

   Multiple admissions are a sign that disease-modifying treatment is inadequate to control symptoms, relieve suffering, or prevent decline in function.

4. Objective measures of functional decline include increasing dependence in Activities of Daily Living, unintentional weight loss, and decreasing albumin level.

5. The palliative response to debility includes symptom management, advance directive discussion, assessment of eligibility for hospice care, and truth-telling with patient and family.

   A palliative-care consult may be helpful to meld symptom management with disease-modifying treatment.

Debility

The Palliative

Response

General Debility
Definition

- Declining functional status with limited prognosis

- Condition may include multiple medical problems

- None of medical conditions necessarily terminal on its own

Know Signs of Life's End

While no one knows how long anyone will live, there are certain signs that health is very poor and declining and time could be limited

Palliative Evaluation
of Suffering in Debility

- Physical
  Poorly controlled physical symptoms (e.g., pain, anorexia, asthenia)

- Emotional
  Distress in the face of physical decline

Palliative Evaluation
of Suffering in Debility

- Social
  Distress from need for additional supportive services

- Spiritual/Existential
  Existential angst
  Feeling of hopelessness

Palliative Response
Overview

- Symptom management
  Development of plan of care to palliate symptoms not relieved by disease-modifying treatment
- Advance directive discussion
  Document surrogate decision maker(s)
  Educate and guide about treatment preferences
  Appropriate in any debilitating illness
- Assess eligibility for hospice referral
- Truth-telling to patient and family

Prognostication
Value to Patient/Family

- Aids in symptom management
- Allows time to access community resources
- Fosters preparing and planning care
- Helps avoid lurching from crisis to crisis

Determining Prognosis

- Can be difficult in individual case
- "Would I be surprised if patient died in the next six months?"

yields a more accurate answer than

"Will this patient die in next six months?"

If you would not be surprised, assess palliative care needs

Language Is Important

"Because of the severity of your illness, you and your family are eligible for the assistance of hospice at home"

is preferable to

"You have a prognosis of less than six months; therefore, I am referring you to hospice"

Example of Life-Limiting Illness

- Combination of diagnoses in 84-year-old
  Moderately severe dementia
  Progressive heart failure
  Chronic renal disease
- Status despite medical management
  Unintentional weight loss
  Confined to bed
- Patient and/or family choose palliation
  Relief of symptoms and suffering vs. cure

Markers for Poor Prognosis in Debility

- Disease progression
  Of one or more of underlying diseases
  Although none yet considered terminal
- Increased dependence
- Need for home-care services

Markers for Poor Prognosis in Debility

- Multiple Emergency Room visits
- Multiple hospital admissions are signs that disease-modifying treatment is inadequate to:
  Control symptoms
  Relieve suffering
  Prevent decline in function

Functional Decline
Objective Measures

- Activities of Daily Living (ADL)
  Development of dependence in at least three ADLs in the last six months:
  Bathing
  Dressing
  Feeding
  Transfers
  Continence
  Ability to walk unaided to the bathroom

Functional Decline
Objective Measures

- Karnofsky performance status
  Karnofsky Score (KS) 50% or less with decline in score over last 6 months
- KS 70%
  Cares for self
  Unable to carry on normal activity or active work
- KS 50%
  Requires considerable assistance
  Requires frequent medical care

Functional Decline
Objective Measures

- Unintentional weight loss
  Greater than or equal to 10% of body weight in the last 6 months

- Albumin
  Less than 2.5 mg/dl
  Always combine this measure with other evidence of decline

Palliative Care Consult
Indications

- Unrelieved suffering

- Functional decline
  Any combination of measures of decline or markers for poor prognosis

- Consideration of hospice referral

Palliative Care Consult
Value

- Symptom control
  Assessment
  Plan
- Treatment planning
  Assist to define Goals of Care
  Assist to develop plan that melds symptom management with disease-modifying treatment
- Assist with advance care planning
- Determine eligibility for hospice care

Palliative Care
in General Debility

Consult often and early.

Debility

Selected Readings

Overview of Debility

Appleton, M. "End-Stage Debility unspecified." *American Journal of Hospice and Palliative Care* 19 (2002): 233–234.

Hamerman, D. "Toward an Understanding of Frailty." *Annals of Internal Medicine* 130 (1999): 945–950.

Kinzbrunner, B. M., N. J. Weinreb , and M. P. Merriman. "Debility, Unspecified: A Terminal Diagnosis." *American Journal of Hospice and Palliative Care* 12 (1996): 38–44.

Resuscitation in the Frail Elderly

Torian, L. V., E. J. Davidson, H. M. Fillit, G. Fulop, and L. L. Sell. "Decisions For and Against Resuscitation in an Acute Geriatric Medicine Unit Serving the Frail Elderly." *Archives of Internal Medicine* 152 (1992): 561–565, erratum on 1659.

1.17 Dementia

Key Points

1. Dementia causes suffering.
    Both patients and their families suffer with physical, spiritual, emotional, and social distress.

2. Dementia requires defining Goals of Care.
    An important role for physicians is to help patients and families define Goals of Care and develop plans for the future.

3. Key markers of advanced dementia indicate referral for hospice care.
    Key markers include inability to walk independently, fewer than six intelligible words, and decline in oral intake.

4. Palliative care is an appropriate treatment philosophy for most patients with dementia.
    A subset of patients with advanced dementia will be eligible to use the Medicare hospice benefit.

5. Housestaff often encounter patients in crisis indicative of complications of late dementia.
    Frequently the crisis indicates the need to change location of care (i.e., home to nursing home).

6. Care of dementia patients should include advance care planning.
    Advance care planning can help patient and family regain a sense of control and reduce suffering and conflict during times of crisis.

Dementia

The Palliative Response

Dementia Causes Suffering

- Physical
- Emotional
- Social
- Spiritual

Both the person afflicted with dementia and the person's family will experience suffering in any or all of these domains

Dementia and Palliative Care

- Most patients and families living with dementia would benefit from the palliative-care approach to the assessment and treatment of their suffering

- Suffering has multiple domains and is best addressed in an interdisciplinary process

Dementia and Hospice Care

A select subset of all patients with dementia will qualify for services through the Medicare hospice benefit.

The Physician's Role

- Evaluation and diagnosis of dementia
- Search for reversible causes (rare)
- Management of current medical problems
- Sensitive revelation of the diagnosis and prognosis
- Assist in defining Goals of Care

The Physician's Role
Medical Management

- Management of acute, often recurrent and infectious illnesses
  Pneumonia
  UTI

- Management of co-morbid illness
  Treatment may be more difficult, especially in the advanced stages of dementia

The Physician's Role
Late-Stage Dementia

- Evaluation of key markers of late-stage dementia

  Inability to walk independently

  Fewer than six intelligible words

  Decline in oral intake and nutritional status

  Frequent ER visits and hospital admission

- Management of late-stage dementia
- Transition to hospice care

Dementia: Physical Suffering

Pain

- Pain from complications of dementia is often undertreated due to difficulty with self-reporting

Infections

- Pneumonia

  Aspirations and atelectasis

- UTI

  Diapers and indwelling catheters

Dementia: Physical Suffering

Decubitis ulcers

- Incontinence
- Immobility
- Restraints
- Poor hygiene
- Decreasing nutritional status

Dementia: Physical Suffering

Asthenia

- Falls
- Bed or chair confinement
- Medical interventions and iatrogenic injury

  Nasogastric tubes and PEG tubes

  Foley catheters

  IVs

  Restraints to protect other interventions or to prevent attempts to get up

Dementia: Emotional Suffering

Depression

- May benefit from treatment with SSRI

Cognitive loss

- May benefit from treatment with medications like donepezil (Aricept) in early-to-moderate stages
- May cause unacceptable side effects without benefit

Dementia: Emotional Suffering

Delirium

- Wandering and sun-downing
- Often worsened by even a minor illness
- Disturbance of sleep-wake cycle disrupts home
- Usually less intense in familiar environments

Dementia: Caregiver Suffering

- Depression
  Referral for treatment
- Fatigue
  Respite
- Anger
  Support groups
- Guilt
  Spiritual counsel/ support groups

Dementia: Social Suffering

- Loss of independence
- Family struggles with role reversal
- Declining health or death of spouse complicates care
- Loss of financial resources
- Need to change location of care

Dementia: Social Suffering

Need to change location of care

- Living at home alone
- Assistance in home
- Living with others
- Assisted-living facility (ALF)
- Nursing home

Dementia: Spiritual Suffering

- Guilt
- Anger
- Inability to maintain relationship with faith community
- Feelings of abandonment

Advance Care Planning
in Early Dementia

Patient can help make decisions

- Surrogates for decision-making
- Preferred locations of care
- Feeding tubes
- Resuscitation and other aggressive interventions

Advance Care Planning
in Advanced Dementia

Family and caregivers discuss decisions

- Transitions to other venues of care
- Response to complications and progression of illness
- Feeding tubes
- Resuscitation attempts

Prognosis

Prediction by fast scoring

- Development of incontinence
  Usually will require transfer from ALF to nursing home

- FAST Score of 6 or 7
  May predict a less than six-month survival
  Qualifies patient for referral to hospice

Prognosis

Key indicators for limited prognosis

- Loss of ability to ambulate independently
- Fewer than six intelligible words
- Declining oral intake

Prognosis

Key indicators for limited prognosis

- Markers of advanced dementia predict
  Frequent ER visits
  Frequent hospital admissions

Prognosis

Key indicators for limited prognosis

- Markers should prompt:
  Discussion with surrogates of limited prognosis
  Review or development of Advance care plan
  Consideration of hospice referral

Dementia

Selected Readings

Life Expectancy

Wolfson, C., D. B. Dolfson, M. Asgharian, C. E. L'Lan, T. Ostbye, D. K. Bockwood, and D. B. Hogan. "A Reevaluation of the Duration of Survival after the Onset of Dementia." *New England Journal of Medicine* 344 (2002): 1111–1116.

Advance Care Planning

Marin, D. B., E. Rudin, B. Fox, J. Neugroschl, A. Brickman, J. Northrop, E. Fine, G. Zaklad, R. S. Morrison, and D. E. Meier. "Feasibility of a Health-Care Proxy Counseling Program for Patients with Alzheimer's Disease." *Journal of Palliative Medicine* 2 (1999): 323–329.

Health Care for Advanced Dementia

Ahronheim, J. C., R. S. Morrison, S. A. Baskin, J. Morris, and D. E. Meier. "Treatment of the Dying in the Acute Care Hospital: Advanced Dementia and Metastatic Cancer." *Archives of Internal Medicine* 156 (1996): 2094–2097.

Luchine, D. J. and P. Hanrahan. "What Is Appropriate Health Care of End-stage Dementia?" *Journal of the American Geriatrics Society* 41 (1993): 25–30.

Tube Feeding

Meier, D. E., J. C. Alronheim, J. Morris, S. Baskin-Lyons, and R. S. Morrison. "High Short-term Mortality in Hospitalized Patients with Advanced Dementia: Lack of Benefit of Tube Feeding." *Archives of Internal Medicine* 161 (2002): 594–599.

Communication

Thompson, P. M. "Communicating with Dementia Patients on Hospice." *American Journal of Hospice and Palliative Care* 19 (2002): 263–266.

Nursing-Home Placement

Yaffe, K., P. Fox, R. Newcomer, L. Sands, K. Lindquist, K. Dane, and K. E. Covinsky. "Patient and Caregiver Characteristics and Nursing Home Placement in Patients with Dementia." *Journal of the American Medical Association* 287 (2002): 2090–2097.

1.18 Progressive Liver Disease

Key Points

1. End-stage liver diseases share many of the same symptoms and general guidelines for predicting prognosis.

    End-stage liver diseases, marked by hepatic insufficiency and cirrhosis, can arise from a variety of specific diagnoses.

2. Palliative-care response includes symptom management, Advance care planning, truth-telling and prognostication, and assessment for hospice care.

    Advance care planning is appropriate for any patient with end-stage liver disease. Truth-telling assists with symptom management and enables patient to access community resources, prepare for dying, and prevent lurching from crisis to crisis.

3. Multiple ER visits and hospital admissions can serve as a trigger for prognostication.

    These events are typical of patients with end-stage liver disease and indicate poorly controlled symptoms.

4. It is important to share the prognosis with the patient and family.

    Choice of language is very important. "Because of the severity of your disease, you and your family are eligible for the assistance of hospice at home" is preferable to "You have a prognosis of less than six months; therefore, I am referring you to hospice."

5. Assess patient's appropriateness and preference for liver transplant.

    Patients and families not pursuing liver transplant may elect to direct Goals of Care and treatment to relief of symptoms and suffering rather than to cure of underlying diseases.

6. Palliative-care consultation can assist with evaluation, treatment, and ongoing management of unrelieved suffering.

    Consider a palliative consultation to assist with assessing symptom control, advising about Goals of Care and development of treatment plan, melding symptom management with disease-modifying treatment, advance care planning, and evaluation of appropriateness/eligibility for hospice care.

Progressive Liver Disease

The Palliative Response

End-Stage Liver Diseases

- Markers
  Hepatic insufficiency
  Cirrhosis
- Etiology
  Can arise from various specific diagnoses
- Symptoms
  Share many of the same symptoms
- Prognosis
  Share general guidelines for predicting prognosis

Palliative Care Response
Evaluation

- Physical
  Assess for poorly controlled symptoms (e.g., pain, anorexia, asthenia)
- Emotional
  Distress secondary to physical decline
- Social
  Distress secondary to increased debility
  Need for additional support services
- Existential/Spiritual angst
  Hopelessness secondary to prognosis

Palliative Care Response
Management

- Symptom management
  Develop plan of care to palliate symptoms not relieved by disease-modifying treatment
- Advance care planning
  Discuss choice of surrogate decision-maker(s)
  Inform and guide regarding treatment preferences
  Any patient with end-stage liver disease needs to document surrogate(s) and preferences

Palliative Care Response
Truth-Telling and Referral

- Truth-telling/prognostication
  Assists with symptom management
  Enables access of community resources
  Facilitates preparing and planning care
  Prevents lurching from crisis to crisis
- Assess eligibility for hospice care

Triggers for Prognostication

- Multiple Emergency Room visits

- Multiple hospital admissions
  Typical of patients with hepatic failure
  Indicate poorly controlled symptoms

Determining Prognosis

Determining individual prognosis is difficult

"Would I be surprised if this patient died in next six months?"

yields more accurate prognosis than

"Will this patient die in the next six months?"

If you would not be surprised, assess palliative needs

Sharing Prognosis

Important for people to know that prognosis is limited

- "While no one knows how long anyone will live, there are certain signs that your health is very poor and declining and that time could be limited"

- "People are eligible for hospice when their illness is so severe that they might die in the next six months to a year"

Language Is Important

"Because of the severity of your disease, you and your family are eligible for the assistance of hospice at home"

is preferable to

"You have a prognosis of less than six months; therefore, I am referring you to hospice"

Is Patient a Candidate for Liver Transplant?

If YES:
- Pursue aggressive treatment goals

Is Patient a Candidate for Liver Transplant?

If NO (due to ineligibility or choice):

- Patient and/or family may elect palliative care
  After discussion with physicians
  Direct Goals of Care and treatment to relief of symptoms and suffering rather than to cure of underlying diseases

Markers for Poor Prognosis
Synthetic Function Impairment

- Severe synthetic function impairment
  Serum Albumin less than 2.5gm/dl
  Prolonged INR greater than 2.0

- Indications to assess for improvement
  Acute illness resolves
  Abstinence from alcohol

Markers for Poor Prognosis
Clinical Indicators

- Refractory ascites

  Lack of response to diuretics
  Nonadherence to treatment

- Spontaneous bacterial peritonitis

- Hepatorenal syndrome

Markers for Poor Prognosis
Clinical Indicators

- Recurrent hepatic encephalopathy

  Decreased response to treatment
  Nonadherence to treatment

- Recurrent variceal bleeding

  Despite medical intervention and management

Other Markers for Poor Prognosis

- Unintentional weight loss
  Greater than or equal to 10% of body weight In the last 6 months
- Muscle wasting/reduced strength
- Continued alcohol use
- HBsAg positivity
- Multiple ER and hospital admissions

Consider
Palliative Care Consult

- <u>Any combination</u> of markers for poor prognosis

- Not necessary for patient to have all signs or symptoms

Palliative Care Consult

- Unrelieved suffering
  Assess symptom control
  Advise about Goals of Care
  Assist to meld symptom management with disease- modifying treatment
- Advance care planning
- Evaluate for hospice referral
  Help establish life-expectancy
  Determine eligibility for hospice care

Palliative Care and Progressive Liver Disease

Consult often and early.

Selected Readings

Management of Ascites

Bui, C. D. H., C. J. Martin, and D. C. Currow. "Effective Community Palliation of Intractable Malignant Ascites with a Permanently Implanted Abdominal Drain." *Journal of Palliative Medicine* 2 (1999): 319–321.

Iyengar, T. D. and T. J. Herzog. "Management of Symptomatic Ascites in Recurrent Ovarian Cancer Patients Using an Intra-abdominal Semi-permanent Catheter." *American Journal of Hospice and Palliative Care* 19 (2002): 35–38.

Management of Variceal Hemorrhage

Sharara, A. I. and D. C. Rockey. "Gastroesophageal Variceal Hemorrhage." *New England Journal of Medicine* 345 (2001): 669–679.

Management of Complications of Cirrhosis

McGuire, B. M. and J. R. Bloomer. "Complication of Cirrhosis: Why They Occur and What to Do about Them." *Postgraduate Medicine* 102 (1998): 209–223.

1.19 Pulmonary Disease

Key Points

1. Palliative evaluation includes assessment of physical, emotional, social, and spiritual suffering.

   Evaluate for uncontrolled physical symptoms such as dyspnea and asthenia; for emotional distress secondary to physical decline; social distress secondary to debility and need for additional support and services; and spiritual distress in the form of existential angst and hopelessness.

2. The palliative response includes managing symptoms, assisting with advance directive and hospice referral, and prognostication and truth-telling.

   Managing symptoms includes developing a plan of care to palliate symptoms unrelieved by disease-modifying treatment. Advance planning includes discussing choice of surrogate decision maker(s) and treatment preferences.

3. Prognostication and truth-telling is valuable to treatment process and to patient/family planning.

   Truth-telling about prognosis assists with symptom management, enables doctor/patient/family to access community resources, fosters preparing and planning care, and helps families avoid lurching from crisis to crisis.

4. Disabling dyspnea is a marker for poor prognosis in advanced pulmonary disease.

   Disabling dyspnea is dyspnea at rest despite maximum medical management. Patients may be very limited (e.g., bed-to-chair or mostly bed confined), and other problems often present (e.g., cough, profound fatigue). Consider co-morbid illnesses.

5. Functional markers for poor prognosis include multiple Emergency Room visits and hospital admissions, declining functional status based on assessment of activities of daily living (ADL), and inability to live independently.

6. There are five key clinical markers for poor prognosis in pulmonary disease:

   Weight loss greater than or equal greater than 10% of body weight over six months; resting tachycardia greater than 100 heart beats/minute; hypoxemia at rest despite supplemental oxygen, such as 21 NP; hypercapnia or pCO2 greater than or equal to 50mm HG; and evidence of right heart failure.

Pulmonary Disease

The Palliative Response

Suffering in Pulmonary Disease

Patients with advanced pulmonary disease often suffer extensively despite maximum disease-modifying therapies.

Palliative Care Evaluation

Physical discomfort

- Poorly controlled symptoms (e.g., dyspnea and asthenia)

Emotional distress
- Secondary to physical decline

Palliative Care Evaluation

Social distress
- Secondary to debility and need for additional support and services

Spiritual distress
- Existential angst and hopelessness

Palliative Care Response
Manage symptoms
- Develop plan to palliate symptoms unrelieved by disease-modifying treatment

Discuss advance directive
- Discuss choice of surrogate decision maker(s)
- Discuss treatment preferences
- Appropriate in any advanced pulmonary disease

Evaluate for hospice referral

Palliative Care Response
Prognostication

Value of truth-telling
- Assists with symptom management
- Enables patient and family to access community resources
- Fosters preparing and planning care
- Helps family avoid lurching from crisis to crisis

Aids to Prognostication

- Determining individual prognosis is difficult
- "Would I be surprised if this patient died in the next six months?"

yields more accurate answer than

"Will this patient die in the next six months?"

If you would not be surprised, assess for palliative care needs

Language Is Important

"Because of the severity of your lung disease, you and your family are eligible for the assistance of hospice at home"

is preferable to

"You have a prognosis of less than six months. Therefore, I am referring you to hospice"

Language Is Important

- "While no one knows how long anyone will live, there are certain signs that your lung disease is very severe and that time could be limited"

- "People are eligible for hospice when their illness is so severe that they might die in the next six months to a year"

Markers for Poor Prognosis
Disabling Dyspnea

- Dyspnea at rest despite maximum medical management
- Patients may be very limited (e.g., bed-to-chair or mostly bed confined)
- Other problems often present (e.g., cough, profound fatigue)
- Consider co-morbid illnesses

Poor Prognosis
Functional Markers

- Multiple Emergency Room visits
- Multiple hospital admissions
- Declining functional status (based on assessment of activities of daily living)
- Inability to live independently (necessitating move to live with family or in a residential care facility)

Poor Prognosis
Five Key Clinical Markers

1. Unintentional weight loss

- Greater than 10% of body weight
- Over six months

Poor Prognosis
Five Key Clinical Markers

2. Resting tachycardia
- Resting heart beat >100/minute
- Unrelated to recent breathing treatment
- Unrelated to atrial fibrillation
- Unrelated to MAT

Poor Prognosis
Five Key Clinical Markers

3. Hypoxemia at rest
- Despite supplemental oxygen, such as 2l NP, pO2 less than or equal to 55mm HG

4. Hypercapnia
- pCO2 greater than or equal to 50mm HG

Poor Prognosis
Five Key Clinical Markers

5. Evidence of right heart failure
- Physical Signs of RHF
- Echocardiogram
- Electrocardiogram

Palliative Care Evaluation
Indication

- Any combination of markers of poor prognosis warrants referral for palliative-care evaluation

- Not necessary or appropriate for patient to exhibit all markers to warrant palliative evaluation

Palliative Care Consult
Review of Contribution

- Unrelieved suffering
  Assess symptom control
  Assist to develop treatment plan that melds symptom management with disease-modifying treatment
- Goals of Care
- Advance care planning
- Assess for hospice referral

Palliative Care and Pulmonary Disease

Consult often and early.

Pulmonary Disease

Selected Readings

Symptom Frequency and Severity

Lutz, S., R. Norrell, C. Bertucio, L. Kachnic et al. "Symptom Frequency and Severity in Patients with Metastatic or Locally Recurrent Lung Cancer: A Prospective Study Using the Lung Cancer Symptom Scale in a Community Hospital." *Journal of Palliative Medicine* 4 (2001): 157–165.

Palliative Care

Gore, J. M., C. J. Brophy, and M. A. Greenstone. "How Well Do We Care for Patients with End Stage Chronic Obstructive Pulmonary Disease (COPD)? A comparison of Palliative Care and Quality of Life in COPD and Lung Cancer." *Thorax* 55 (2000): 1000–1006.

Skilbeck, J., L. Mott, H. Page, D. Smith, S. Hjelmeland-Ahmedzai, and D. Clark. "Palliative Care in Chronic Obstructive Airways Disease: A Needs Assessment." *Palliative Medicine* 12 (1998): 245–254.

Hospice Care

Abrahm, J. L. and J. Hansen-Flaschen. "Hospice Care for Patients with Advanced Lung Disease." *Chest* 121 (2002): 220–229.

1.20 Renal Disease

Key Points

1. Patients with end-stage renal disease often suffer extensively despite maximum disease-modifying therapies.

    Some patients decline or discontinue dialysis therapy; others are inappropriate because of co-morbid diseases or Quality-of-Life issues.

2. Evaluate patients with end-stage renal disease for suffering in the physical, emotional, social and spiritual realms.

    Evaluate for uncontrolled physical symptoms such as dyspnea, asthenia and delirium; emotional distress in the face of physical decline; social distress from increased debility and need for additional services; and spiritual distress in the form of existential angst and hopelessness.

3. The palliative response to end-stage renal disease includes symptom management and advanced planning:

    Symptom management includes developing a plan to palliate symptoms unrelieved by disease-modifying treatment. Advance directive planning includes discussions with the patient to choose surrogate decision-maker(s) and determine treatment preferences.

4. Truth-telling assists with symptom management, enables accessing community resources, fosters preparing and planning care, and helps the patient and family avoid lurching from crisis to crisis.

5. There are key clinical markers for end-stage renal disease.

    Clinical markers include weight loss greater than 10% of body weight over the previous six months, and resting tachycardia of heartbeat greater than 100/minute unrelated to recent breathing treatment, atrial fibrillation, or MAT. Important laboratory markers indicating poor prognosis for patients not to be dialyzed are serum creatinine >8mg/dl and creatinine clearance <10cc/minute.

6. Functional markers of poor prognosis include multiple Emergency Room visits and hospital admissions and declining functional status based on assessment of ADL and ability to live independently.

7. Any combination of markers for poor prognosis might prompt evaluation by palliative care for unrelieved suffering or for hospice referral.

Renal Disease

The Palliative Response

Suffering in End-Stage Renal Disease

Patients with end-stage renal disease often suffer extensively despite maximum disease-modifying therapies.

Dialysis Therapy

- Some patients decline
- Some patients inappropriate
  Co-morbid diseases
  Quality-of-Life issues
- Some patients decide to discontinue
  Progressive decline
  Co-morbid illness
  Appropriate for hospice referral

Palliative Evaluation

- Physical
  Uncontrolled symptoms (e.g., Dyspnea, Asthenia, Delirium)

- Emotional
  Distress in the face of physical decline

Palliative Evaluation

- Social
  Distress from increased debility and need for additional services

- Spiritual
  Existential angst and hopelessness

The Palliative Response

- Symptom management
  Develop plan of care to palliate symptoms not relieved by disease-modifying treatment
- Advance directive discussion
  Discuss surrogate decision maker(s)
  Discuss treatment preferences
  Document result of discussion
- Hospice referral for advanced patients
- Truth-telling

Value of Truth-Telling and Prognostication

- Assists with symptom management
- Enables accessing community resources
- Fosters preparing and planning care
- Helps avoid lurching from crisis to crisis

Establishing Prognosis

"Would you be surprised if this patient died in next six months?"

Yields more accurate prognosis than...

"Will this patient die in the next six months?"

If you would not be surprised, assess for palliative care needs.

Sharing Prognosis
Important for people to know that prognosis is limited

"Because of the severity of your kidney disease, you and your family are eligible for the assistance of hospice at home"

is preferable to...

"You have a prognosis of less than six months; therefore, I am referring you to hospice"

Language Is Important

- "While no one knows how long anyone will live, there are certain signs that your kidney disease is very severe and that time could be limited"

- "People are eligible for hospice when their illness is so severe that they might die in the next six months to a year"

Markers for Poor Prognosis
Co-Morbid Illnesses

- Strokes
- Advanced dementia
- Congestive heart failure despite control of fluid overload

Markers for Poor Prognosis
Co-Morbid Illnesses

- Chronic lung disease
  Oxygen dependence

- Diabetes mellitus
  Manifestations of long-term complications

Poor Prognosis
Key Clinical Markers

- Unintentional weight loss
  Greater than 10% of body weight over six months
- Resting tachycardia
  Resting heartbeat greater than 100/ minute
  Unrelated to recent breathing treatment, atrial fibrillation, or MAT

Poor Prognosis
Key Clinical Markers

Poor prognostic markers for patient who will not be receiving dialysis

- Serum Creatinine >8mg/dl
- Creatinine Clearance <10cc/ minute

Poor Prognosis
Functional Markers

- Multiple Emergency Room visits
- Multiple hospital admissions
- Declining functional status based on assessment of activities of daily living
- Need to move from living independently to living with family or in a residential-care facility

Palliative Response to
Markers for Poor Prognosis

- Any combination of markers for poor prognosis might prompt evaluation by palliative care for unrelieved suffering or for hospice referal

- It is not necessary or appropriate for a patient to exhibit all of the markers before being evaluated by palliative care

Palliative Care Consult

- Symptom control
- Treatment plan
  Assist to develop plan that melds symptom management with disease-modifying treatment
- Goals of Care
- Advance care planning
- Assess for hospice care

Palliative Care
End-Stage Renal Disease

Consult often and early.

Renal Disease

Selected Readings

Withdrawing Dialysis

Choen, L. M., M. J. Germain, D. M. Poppel, A. L. Woods, P. S. Pekow, and C. M. Kjellstrand. "Dying Well after Discontinuing the Life-support Treatment of Dialysis." *Archives of Internal Medicine* 160 (2000); 2513–2518.

Neely, K. J. and D. M. Roxe. "Palliative Care/Hospice and the Withdrawal of Dialysis." *Journal of Palliative Medicine* 3 (2000): 57–67.

Quality of Dying

Cohen, L. M., D. M. Poppel, G. M. Cohn, and G. S. Reiter. "A Very Good Death: Measuring Quality of Dying in End-stage Renal Disease." *Journal of Palliative Medicine* 4 (2001): 167–172.

Association with Myocardial Infarction

Shlipak, M. G., P. A. Heidenreich, H. Noguchi, G. M. Chertow et al. "Association of Renal Insuffieiency with Treatment and Outcomes after Myocardial Infarction in Elderly Patients." *Annals of Internal Medicine* 137 (2002): 555–562.

1.21 Congestive Heart Failure

Key Points

1. Congestive heart failure (CHF) includes physical, social, emotional, and spiritual suffering.

2. All forms of suffering and distress affect the Quality of Life (QOL).
   Fewer than half of respondents rate QOL as good. Loss of function, low mood, mental confusion, and incontinence are predictive of poor QOL. Pain and dyspnea, while contributing to poor QOL, are not as predictive.

3. Data about dying from CHF come from retrospective and prospective studies and clinical experience.
   Results reveal that 2 of 3 patients experience one or more difficult-to-tolerate physical or emotional symptoms. Family reports indicate that 59% of patients would have preferred a palliative approach and that, in 10% of patients, some aspect of care was contrary to stated wishes.

4. Survival in CHF patients is variable and hard to predict.
   Poor prognostic signs are lower systolic BP, elevated creatinine, and persistent rales. Attempts to predict survival contribute to unrelieved suffering by depriving many patients of palliative management since they are not deemed six months from death.

5. The palliative approach to caring for CHF patients is comprehensive and holistic.
   Palliative care for CHF focuses on symptom management rather than disease modification. Interventions include psychological, emotional and bereavement support; care of the family; access to community resources; interdisciplinary teaching; home services; and advance care planning.

6. Communication problems are common between CHF patients and physicians.
   Communication problems may be due to patient confusion and short-term memory loss, difficulty of prediction, or physicians' discomfort about addressing key concerns openly and frankly.

Congestive Heart Failure

The Palliative Response

Dying from Heart Disease
Physical Suffering at Life's End

- PAIN was one of the most common problems
- 78% report pain in the last year
- 63% report pain in the last week
- 50% say pain is "very distressing"

- DYSPNEA was the second most common problem
- 61% report dyspnea in the last year
- 51% report dyspnea in the last week
- 43% say dyspnea is "very distressing"

McCarthy et. al., 1996

Dying from Heart Disease
Physical Suffering at Life's End

- Loss of appetite   43%
- Nausea/vomiting   32%
- Constipation   37%
- Fecal incontinence   16%

McCarthy et al, 1996

Dying from Heart Disease
Physical Suffering at Life's End

- Low mood   59%
- Sleeplessness 45%
- Anxiety   30%
- Mental confusion
  Under age 55   27%
  Over age 85   42%

  Much more distressing for younger than older patients

McCarthy et al, 1996

Social and Spiritual Suffering
at Life's End

- Dying in setting other than home (70%)
- Declining functional status
- Social isolation
- Depletion of financial resources
- Caregiver fatigue
- Questions of meaning – Why?

Predictors
of Poor Quality of Life (QOL)

- Loss of function
- Low mood
- Mental confusion
- Incontinence
- Pain/dyspnea contribute but less predictive

*All forms of suffering reduce QOL
Fewer than half report good QOL at Life's End*

Status and Symptoms
at Life's End

- 55% conscious in the last three days
- 4 of 10 had severe pain most of the time
- 8 of 10 had severe asthenia
- 1 of 4 had severe dysphoria
- 2 of 3 had one or more difficult-to-tolerate physical or emotional symptoms

Interventions
at Life's End

- 11%—final resuscitation event
- 25%—ventilator support
- 40%—feeding tube
- 59%—would have preferred comfort care (as reported by family)
- 10%—some aspect of care was contrary to stated wishes

Congestive Heart Failure
Survival Study

Time in Months	Survival
1	81%
3	75%
6	70%
12	62%
18	57%

Poor Prognostic Signs
Lower Systolic BP—Elevated Creatinine
Persistent Rales

Cowie et al, 2000

Six-Month Survival Rates
Congestive Heart Failure

- Ejection fraction <20%   73%
- Arhythmia   75%
- Inclusion to hospice
  - Broad 473   75%
  - Intermediate 170   69%
  - Narrow 12   58%

Lynn et al, 1999

Congestive Heart Failure
Survival Can Be Unpredictably Short

- Impossible to predict accurately which congestive heart patients will die in given period
- Many patients die before judged "eligible" for hospice care by their predicted life expectancy
- Thus, many patients amenable to palliative care instead experience unrelieved suffering

SUPPORT Study
Lynn et al, 1999

Congestive Heart Failure
The Palliative Response

- Symptom management (vs. disease modification)
- Psychological, emotional, and bereavement support
- Care of the family unit
- Access to community resources
- Interdisciplinary assistance
- Home services
- Advance care planning

Doctor–Patient Communication
about Death and Dying

Evidence of communication difficulty
- Many patients realized they were dying, but without any input from physician about this reality
- Patients queried researchers about condition, prognosis, and likely manner of death

Etiology of communication difficulty
- Patients—confusion, memory loss
- Physicians—discomfort, unwillingness to provide information

Optimum Medical Treatment

- Ace inhibitors
- Digoxin
- Loop diuretics
- Beta-blockers
- Spironolactone
- Anticoagulant therapy
- Nitrates

Breathlessness

- KEEP DRY, reposition, reassure, provide a fan
- Oxygen
- Morphine or another opioid in short-acting form
  Ms 10mg/5ml 5–10mg q1–2 hour for dyspnea
- Mild anxiolytic
  Lorazepam 0.5–1mg q2–4 hours
- Relief of dyspnea is more important than determining the creatinine level

Diuretic Treatment Is Key in Breathlessness
Goals
- Minimal rales and patient comfort
- Weight control
  Weigh and chart daily
  If weight increases, increase diuretics/reduce fluid intake
  If weight decreases, reduce diuretic until weight stabilizes

Possible unavoidable side effects
- Hypotension
- Elevated creatinine and BUN
- Dry mouth

Home Nursing Role

- Assist with medicines
- Assist with diet
- Assist with memory
- Assess patient safety and comfort
  Bed or recliner with raised head?
  Easy access to toilet
  Family support
  Need for additional assistance (home health aides, homemaker, meals)

Fatigue and Lightheadedness

- Reassess drug therapy
- Consider depression
- Recommend energy conservation
- Check for postural hypotension
- If dyspnea is controlled, may be able to titrate fluid intake to increase intravascular volume with oral hydration

Nausea and Anorexia

Etiology

- Complications of drug therapy
- Constipation secondary to medicines or decreased fluid intake

Interventions

- Frequent small meals to accommodate fatigue
- Appetite stimulant (e.g., alcohol or decadron)
- Metoclopramide for decreased emptying

Edema

Interventions

- Diuretic therapy
- Fluid restriction
- Elevation
- Salt restriction
- Reassurance

Consider Etiology

- Anasarca
- Decreased albumin level

Emotional Suffering

Manifestations

- Delirium
- Depression
- Anxiety

Interventions

- Medical management
- Supportive home environment
- Openly address fears to help regain sense of control

Social Suffering

Etiology

- Loss of income
- Cost of treatment
- Difficulty with transportation and errands
- Necessity for residential care vs. home care
- Time limits and lack of defined prognosis

Interventions

- Access community resources

Spiritual Suffering

Etiology

- Uncertainty about timing/manner of death
- Guilt and anger
- Sense of isolation and abandonment due to fatigue of caregivers and other supporters

Intervention

- Improve symptom control
- Reconnect with community

Programmatic Response

- Hospice care in advanced and difficult cases for intensive support
- Congestive heart home health specialist (offered by some insurances)
- Medicaring demonstration project (supportive services for CHF and COPD)

Congestive Heart Failure

Selected Readings

Incidence and Survival

Levy, D., S. Kenchaiah, M. G. Larson et al. "Long-term Trends in the Incidence of and Survival with Heart Failure." *New England Journal of Medicine* 347 (2002): 1397–1402.

Care of the Bereaved

Edwards, L. and D. G. Shaw. "Care of the Suddenly Bereaved in Cardiac Care Units: A Review of the Literature." [Review] [66 refs]. *Intensive and Critical Care Nursing* 14 (1998): 144–152.

1.22 HIV/AIDS (I)

Key Points

1. Protease inhibitors are used widely in both newly infected and established patients.

2. HIV/AIDS is now considered a chronic illness such as diabetes mellitus or hypertension.

3. Physical suffering in HIV/AIDS may come from opportunistic infection, malignancy, treatment toxicity, or organ failure.
   Opportunistic infections may develop when immune competency cannot be restored due to disease resistance, patient noncompliance, or lack of availability of treatment. Opportunistic infections—which include MAC, CMV, toxoplasmosis, and wasting—may lead to death within 12 months of onset.

4. Complications may develop when immune competency cannot be restored.
   Complications include progressive multifocal leukoencephalopathy; dementia; and cancers such as B cell lymphoma, primary CNS lymphoma, and cervical cancer in women. Complications may lead to death within 12 months of onset.

5. Complications may develop from treatment.
   Complications of treatment may include diabetes mellitus, pancreatitis, lipid dystrophy with stroke or heart disease, hepatic injury, or bone marrow suppression.

6. Other complications or organ failures may develop.

HIV-AIDS (II)

Key Points

1. HIV/AIDS often involves significant emotional suffering.
   Emotional suffering of HIV/AIDS hospice patients may include depression and suicidality, cognitive impairment, substance abuse, anxiety, mental illness and homelessness, and issues of gender and sexuality.

2. HIV/AIDS often involves significant social suffering.
   Social suffering of HIV/AIDS hospice patients may be related to relative youth of infected persons; infection of multiple members of family or community group; estrangement from family and/or society; loss of income and lack of insurance; unstable living environment; loneliness and dissatisfaction with available support; lack of recognized long-term relationship; need for advance care planning; and need for residential care.

3. HIV/AIDS often involves significant spiritual suffering.
   Spiritual suffering of HIV/AIDS hospice patients may be related to perceived and/or actual discrimination secondary to sexual expression, race, ethnicity and/or class; perceived and/or actual rejection by faith community; fear of divine judgment and retribution; lack of time to process life events and develop sources of meaning and transcendence; and unmet need for grace and mercy.

4. Persons with HIV/AIDS frequently receive care at Life's End in "nontraditional" hospice settings such as acute care hospitals, residential care facilities, and prisons.
   Late hospice referrals are frequent for persons with HIV/AIDS due to patients' hesitation to accept hospice care, providers' difficulty determining appropriateness because of effectiveness of HAART treatment, and absence of stable home environment and primary caregiver.
   New service models incorporating coordinated and holistic interdisciplinary care may be especially important in treating persons with HIV/AIDS, who have met with fear, prejudice, and discrimination in the healthcare system.

5. Palliative care for persons with HIV/AIDS could become a model for incorporation of palliative care into treatment of other chronic illnesses.

HIV/AIDS

The Palliative Response

Changing Natural History
of HIV/AIDS

Early 1980s
Clusters of PCP Pneumonia

- Identification of high-risk groups in US
  Gay men
  Injecting drug users
  Hemophiliacs

Changing Natural History
of HIV/AIDS

Mid 1980s
Identification of HIV as the causative agent

- Screening and testing of at-risk groups
- Identification of the routes of infection
- Development of education/ prevention campaigns
- Mounting numbers of deaths from AIDS

Changing Natural History
of HIV/AIDS

Mid 1980s
Understanding of the natural history of infection

- Acute infection (usually not recognized)
- Long asymptotic (infectious) period
- ARC (AIDS related complex)
- Opportunistic infection and/or certain types of cancers leading to death

---

Changing Natural History
of HIV/AIDS

Mid 1980s
Understanding of the natural history of infection

- Lose about 100 CD4s/year
- Relationship to CD4 lymphocyte depletion

500–1000/dl	*Normal*
200–500/dl	*ARC*
<200/dl	*PCP*
<100/dl	*Other opportunistic infections (OI) and*
death	

Changing Natural History
of HIV/AIDS

Late 1980s
Treatment

- TMP/Sulfa for PCP
- AZT trial
- DDI trial
- People living longer develop other opportunistic infections
  Cytomegalovirus (CMV)
  Mycobacterium Avium Complet (MAC)

Changing Natural History
of HIV/AIDS

Early 1990s
Recognition that the medicines developed could be toxic and lose effectiveness

- Development of other NRTIs
- Development of NNRTIs
- HIV/AIDS hospice programs in larger cities (San Francisco, New York, Chicago)

Changing Natural History
of HIV/AIDS

Early 1990s

- Beginning to appreciate the crisis developing in Sub-Saharan Africa, Asia, and other developing countries
- Hospice programs in smaller communities begin to have more referrals as local infection occurs and persons living with AIDS (PWA) return to live with their families

Changing Natural History
of HIV/AIDS

Early 1990s
Finding expression for the crisis

- AIDS Quilt
- Red Ribbons
- *Angels in America* (play)
- *RENT* (musical)
- *The Band Played On* (book and movie)
- *Philadelphia* (movie)

Changing Natural History
of HIV/AIDS

Early 1990s
New treatments

- PI Protease Inhibitors introduced
- HAART (Highly Active Anti-Retroviral Therapy) 2NRTIs and a PI
- People with AIDS on their death beds got up and walked out of hospices
- Irrational exuberance (possible cure)

Changing Natural History
of HIV/AIDS

Late 1990s to present

- PI Protease Inhibitors widely used in both newly infected and established patients
- HIV/AID specialty hospice programs close
- New side effects and toxicity identified
- Cost of treatment > $1000/month
- Patients begin to fail treatment because of the development of resistance

Changing Natural History
of HIV/AIDS

Late 1990s to present:
Infection escalates
in developing countries

- HIV/AIDS infection rate in some South African countries reaches 25% of the population
- Protest about the inability to afford or access treatment in developing countries
- Development of HIV/AIDS hospice care in developing world

Changing Natural History
of HIV/AIDS

Late 1990s to present

- View HIV/AIDS in USA as chronic illness such as DM or HTN

- Hospice referral of patients with HIV/AIDS resumes

- The future

The Experience of Dying from HIV/AIDS

Social

Physical

Suffering

Emotional

Spiritual

Palliative Care

"Palliative care seeks to prevent, relieve, reduce or soothe the symptoms of disease or disorder without effecting a cure...

Palliative care in this broad sense is not restricted to those who are dying or those enrolled in hospice programs...

It attends closely to the emotional, spiritual, and practical needs and goals of patients and those close to them."

Institute of Medicine 1998

Palliative Care

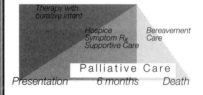

Therapy with curative intent

Hospice
Symptom R$_x$
Supportive Care

Bereavement Care

Palliative Care

Presentation   6 months   Death

Physical Suffering

- Opportunistic infection (OI)
- Malignancy
- Treatment toxicity
- Organ failure

Physical Suffering
Opportunistic Infection

Opportunistic infection may develop when immune competency cannot be restored due to:

- Lack of response (resistance)
- Noncompliance with treatment
- Lack of availability of treatment (developing countries)

Physical Suffering
Opportunistic Infection

Complications when immune-competency cannot be restored may lead to death within 12 months of onset

- MAC   74%
- CMV   70%
- Toxoplasmosis   73%
- CMV and MAC   99%
- CMV and wasting   88%

Physical Suffering
Complications

Complications when immune-competency cannot be restored may lead to death within 12 months of onset

- Progressive multifocal leukoencephalopathy   100%
- Dementia   79%
- Cancers such as B cell lymphoma, primary CNS lymphoma, and cervical cancer in women

Physical Suffering
Complications of Treatment

- Diabetes mellitus
- Pancreatitis
- Lipid dystrophy with stroke or heart disease
- Hepatic injury
- Bone marrow suppression

Physical Suffering
Complications and Organ Failures

- Renal failure
- Liver failure with Hepatitis B and/or C
- Cardiomyopathy
- Co-morbid risk of injury from drug and alcohol abuse

Palliative Care and Hospice Referrals

Indications for referral
- HAART therapy ineffective
- HAART therapy not tolerated well
- PWA declines treatment for HIV
- Complications such as dementia, PML
- HIV may be secondary diagnosis with the primary diagnosis being hepatic failure, cancer, etc.

Palliative and Hospice Care

- Physical symptoms may be similar to those of other patients referred to hospice although may have larger number
- Special issues
  Pain control in patients with history of past or current drug use

  Decisions about continuing some OI or HIV treatments

  Management of specific OI/HIV problems in concert with HIV specialist

Emotional Suffering
and HIV/AIDS

- Depression and suicide
- Cognitive impairment
  Dementia or PML
- Substance abuse
- Anxiety
- Mental illness and homelessness
- Sexuality issues

Social Suffering
and HIV/AIDS

- Relative youth of infected individuals
- Infection of multiple members of family or community group
- Estrangement from family and society
- Loss of income
- Lack of insurance—Medicaid and Medicare issues

Social Suffering
and HIV/AIDS

- Unstable living environment
- Loneliness
- Dissatisfaction with available support
- Lack of recognized long-term relationship
- Need for Advance Care Planning
- Need for residential care

Social Suffering
and HIV/AIDS

Perceived and actual discrimination
- Sexual expression
- Race
- Ethnicity
- Class

Spiritual Suffering
and HIV/AIDS

- Perceived and actual rejection by faith community
- Fear of divine judgment and retribution
- Lack of time to process life events and develop sources of meaning and transcendence
- Unmet need for grace and mercy

Palliative Care
for HIV/AIDS

- Many HIV/AIDS primary care providers have recognized the importance of incorporating nursing, social work, pastoral care, and mental health in a coordinated holistic model of care
- New service models have developed because of fear, prejudice, and discrimination by community providers

Hospice Care
for HIV/AIDS

Late hospice referrals are common
- Difficult for patients to accept hospice
- Difficult for providers to determine appropriateness because of effectiveness of HAART treatment
- Lack of stable home environment and primary caregiver

Hospice Care
for HIV/AIDS

Persons with HIV/AIDS frequently receive EOL care in "nontraditional" hospice settings

- Acute care hospitals
- Residential care facilities
- Prisons

Hospice Care
for HIV/AIDS

- There is an international need for hospice and palliative care as primary treatment because of lack of infrastructure for medical treatment
- HAART is unlikely to become widely available because of expense and difficulty of treatment management in poor and developing countries

Palliative Care
for HIV/AIDS

- Needs to be available to patients and their medical providers
- Could become a model for the incorporation of palliative care into other chronic illnesses
- Care needs to be flexible and responsive to patient and caregiver needs
- Providers need to learn from each other about management of HIV/AIDS throughout the course of the disease

Palliative Care
for HIV/AIDS

Offers possibility for growth

- Individual
- Community
- Profession

HIV/AIDS
and Palliative Care

Consult early and often.

HIV/AIDS

Selected Readings

<u>**Clinical Profile**</u>

Welch, K. et al. "The Clinical Profile of End-stage AIDS. *AIDS Patient Care STDS* 12 (1998): 125–129.

<u>Best Practices of Palliative Care</u>

Arnes, P. J. and I. J. Higginson, "What Constitutes High Quality HIV/AIDS Palliative Care?" *Journal of Palliative Care* 15 (1999): 5–12.

O'Neill, J. F. and C. S. Alexander. "Palliative Medicine and HIV/AIDS." *Primary Care* 24 (1997): 607–615.

O'Neill, J. F., K. Marconi, A. Suprapruik, and N. Blum. "Improving HIV/AIDS Services through Palliative Care: An HRSA Perspective." Health Resources and Services Administration: *Journal of Urban Health* 77 (2000): 244–254.

<u>**Natural History of HIV-AIDS**</u>

Selwyn, P. A. and R. Arnold. "From Fate to Tragedy: The Changing Meanings of Life, Death, and AIDS." *Annals of Internal Medicine* 129: 899–902.

<u>**Spiritual Well-being**</u>

Pace, J. C. and J. L. Stables. "Correlates of Spiritual Well-being in Terminally Ill Persons with AIDS and Terminally Ill Persons with Cancer." *Journal of the Association of Nurses in AIDS Care* 8 (1997): 31–42.

Social Suffering: The Palliative Response

2.1 Access to Medical Care: Medical Insurance and Suffering at Life's End

Key Points

1. Medical insurance or the lack thereof has a major impact on the type of medical care a patient may receive.

   Insurance coverage, rather than patient or family preference, often determines location of care.

2. Many families deplete their savings caring for loved ones at the end-of-life.

   Terminal illness impoverishes 40% of patients and families. Many patients worry about being a financial burden on their families.

3. Private insurance is often contingent on employment. Persons who become ill and unable to work often lose insurance coverage. Private insurance frequently does not cover hospice or home care.

   Payment schedules and covered services vary greatly from policy to policy. Patients who are unable to pay insurance premiums due to illness and loss of income lose their coverage.

4. Medicaid is a federal program administered by the state.

   Patients must apply for Social Security disability to apply for Medicaid.

5. Honorably discharged veterans are eligible for medical services through the Veterans Administration.

   Services and co-payment may vary based on factors such as income and service-connection status.

6. The Medicare hospice benefit covers hospice care.

   A physician certifies an individual as eligible for hospice care based on criteria that reflect the severity of the illness, primarily limited life expectancy. Patients or their representatives sign a form to elect hospice care that is primarily symptom focused and supportive and usually delivered in the home or a nursing home setting.

Access to Medical Care at Life's End

The Palliative Response

Impact of Medical Insurance

- Coverage, or lack thereof, determines

  Type of medical care a patient may receive

  Location of care

- Patients often use several different sources of payment during the course of an illness

Impact of Life's End on Family Finances

- Expenses not covered by insurance
- Loss of income
- Loss of insurance
- Loss of savings
- Loss of assets

Financial Burden

Many additional expenses at Life's End are not covered by insurance

- Transportation
- Medications
- Durable medical supplies
- Nondurable medical supplies
- Co-payments

Loss of Income

- Patient loses job and income due to inability to work
- Family members must leave work or limit hours to care for patient

Loss of Insurance

- Patient loses insurance when unable to maintain employment
- Patient is unable to pay COBRA

  The Consolidated Omnibus Budget Reconciliation Act of 1985 is a law that allows individuals to maintain their insurance if they leave their job. Most are unable to afford the cost if unemployed.

Loss of Savings

- Many families deplete their savings while caring for loved ones at Life's End

Loss of Assets

- Patient often loses home or other assets to qualify for long-term care

Impoverishment

- Terminal illness impoverishes 40% of patients and families

Emotional Burden

- Many patients worry about being a burden on family finances

Forms of Medical Insurance

Medicare

- Part A
- Part B
- Purchase supplements for co-pay
- Medicare HMO

Medicare Hospice Benefit

- Type of care
  - *Primarily symptom management*
  - *Usually delivered in home or nursing home*
- Eligibility
  - *Must have Medicare A*
  - *Physician certifies person as terminally ill and eligible for hospice care*
  - *Patient elects hospice care*
    - *Certifies understanding of terminal status*
    - *Requests care as defined by hospice*

Medicaid

- Administration
  - *Federal program administered by each state*
  - *Differs from state to state*
  - *Funds are a State-Federal match*
- Eligibility
  - *Must first apply for Social Security Disability*
- Primarily covers (e.g., Alabama)
  - *Nursing home care*
  - *Prenatal and obstetrics care*
  - *Pediatric care for children without private insurance*

Veterans Administration

- Eligibility
  - *Honorably discharged veterans*
- Coverage
  - *Services and co-payment may vary*
- Factors determining coverage
  - *Income*
  - *Service-connection status*

Private Insurance

- Policies vary greatly
  - *Payment schedules*
  - *Covered services*
- Limitations for care at Life's End
  - *Hospice or home care frequently not covered*
  - *Patient must continue to pay premiums to maintain coverage*

Medically Indigent

- *Example: Jefferson Health System*
- Eligibility
  - *Medically indigent resident of Jefferson County*
- Coverage
  - *Primary ambulatory and acute hospital care*
  - *Some prescriptions*
  - *Some durable medical supplies*
  - *HOSPICE CARE through County Health Department*
- Co-pay determination
  - *Income*
  - *Size of household*

Access to Medical Care The Palliative Response

- Be aware of realities of healthcare financing
- Be informed about resources available for patients
- Be sensitive to the economic burdens and realities of a life-threatening illness on patients and their families

Case Presentations

Case 1

When Charlie was 40 years old, he began to have severe pain in his left hip that prevented him from working as a construction laborer. Thinking that he had injured himself on the job, he went to see a doctor to explore a worker's compensation claim.

The x-rays revealed that Charlie's problems were much more serious than first believed. He was referred to the oncology clinic, where it was discovered that he had metastatic cancer to the bones from an asymptotic lung cancer in his left lung.

Charlie was informed that:

1. the cancer was incurable because it had spread beyond the lung;
2. his life expectancy was estimated at less than a year (and that patients rarely live more than two years);
3. he would never be able to work again; and
4. he needed to start radiation treatment to reduce the pain in his hip and the risk of fracture, a treatment that would cost approximately $10,000.

Charlie is married with three young children. His employer offered no health insurance benefits.

What would you do?

Options

- Apply for Social Security Disability
  Charlie could wait 3–6 months for a determination.

- Apply for Medicare
  Since Charlie is only 40 years old, he must wait for two years after being deemed disable to apply for Medicare.

- Apply for Medicaid
  Charlie must apply for disability first.

- Apply for Assistance from Local Charities
  Such assistance is usually limited to a one-time benefit of a few hundred dollars.

Charlie is sponsored for the radiation by the local charity hospital. His pain improves, but within three months he develops progressive disease.

Charlie is a candidate for a chemotherapy study for a new experimental drug being compared to standard chemotherapy. Chemotherapy would cost more than $1000 a month. He enrolls in the study, which provides free chemotherapy. One month later, Social Security Disability and Medicaid are granted. Six months later, the lung cancer is stable but the chemotherapy study is completed.

One year after the initial diagnosis, several brain metastases are discovered, and Charlie begins another course of radiation therapy. Charlie enrolls in a hospice program using his Medicaid benefit. Charlie dies 20 months after the original diagnosis and four months before his Medicare benefits were to begin.

Questions

• What are the problems that Charlie had in accessing medical care?

• What are some possible changes in our health-care funding and delivery systems that would have improved Charlie's access to care and the quality of his care?

Case Presentations

Case 2

Brenda, a 35-year-old self-employed cosmetics saleswoman, noticed that she had acquired a pot belly and that, over the last few weeks, she had developed small red spots on her legs. She decided to stop in at a local walk-in emergent care clinic between sales calls. She was told that her platelet count was dangerously low, which might cause her to bleed. Since she had no private insurance, she was referred to the local charity hospital.

Brenda was diagnosed with advanced cirrhosis of the liver brought on by an asymptotic infection with the hepatitis C virus and worsened by daily consumption of 2–3 alcoholic drinks. Further evaluation revealed ascites and an enlarged spleen causing the low platelet count. Brenda also has enlarged veins in her esophagus, called varicies.

Brenda stops drinking any alcohol and begins taking medications to reduce the fluid collection and the chance of a bleeding episode from the varicies. Despite this, she is admitted to the intensive-care unit for a life-threatening bleeding episode that requires more than 8 units of blood.

Brenda and her husband are informed that:

1. the cirrhosis of the liver is irreversible and progressive;
2. only one-third of patients with a bleeding episode survive for one year;
3. a liver transplant might help her condition, but she must have some form of insurance and be abstinent from alcohol for one year before she can be evaluated.

What would you do?

Options

- Apply for Social Security disability
  Brenda could wait 3–6 months for a determination

- Apply for Medicare
  Since Brenda is only 35 years old, she must wait for two years after being deemed disabled to apply for Medicare.

- Apply for Medicaid
  Since Brenda's husband is employed and they have some assets, such as a home and a car of modest value, their income is above the minimum allowed to qualify for Medicaid.

Brenda was awarded Social Security disability three months after the original diagnosis. She has been abstinent for one year but has had two more life-threatening episodes of bleeding and has declining hepatic function. It will be 10 more months before she is eligible for Medicare.

Questions

• What are the problems Brenda had in accessing medical care?

• What are some possible changes in our health-care funding and delivery systems that would have improved Brenda's access to care and the quality of her care?

Case Presentations

Case 3

Despite David'd weight of nearly 325 pounds, his family has managed to bring him to the ER for the third time this month. Each time he received a shot of IV medicine to make him urinate some of the nearly 30 pounds of water weight that had collected since the previous visit and was causing him to gasp for breath.

David had developed severe heart disease secondary to morbid obesity and emphysema from smoking. The ejection fraction of his heart was less than 20% (normal is 60%). David had been intubated in the past when he was severely short of breath and had informed his family and doctor that he wanted no aggressive life support in the future. In light of this and his frequent visits to the ER, David was referred to home hospice.

Having been disabled for more than two years, David qualified for Medicare; but it did not help pay for the expensive medicines required for his heart and lung conditions. The hospice team developed a plan to help David and his family to manage his illness. The plan included setting up David's medications in a pill box, helping the family budget for medicines not covered under the Medicare Hospice Benefit, and daily weighing to adjust David's water pill dose.

In the first month, David controlled his water weight gain, his depression and anxiety improved, the hospice dietician helped him lose nearly 15 pounds, and a low dose of opioid reduced his constant sense of breathlessness and improved his exercise tolerance. After six months with no ER visits, the hospice program discharged David since his prognosis seemed to have improved and was probably greater than the six months required for hospice care.

What would you do?

Outcome

The hospice program tried to prepare David and his family for discharge by establishing him with a primary doctor and seeking financial support for his medicines. David's new doctor did not approve of the use of the opioid (Lortab5™, 1 tablet four times a day) for air hunger, and David found it difficult to keep his clinic appointments.

Four months later, David had three episodes of severe shortness of breath requiring an ER visit. On the third occasion, he died in the ambulance and was coded unsuccessfully.

Questions

• What are the problems that David had in accessing medical care?

• What are some possible changes in our health-care funding and delivery systems that would have improved David's access to care and the quality of his care?

Medicare

Medicare is a national health insurance program for people ≥65 years of age, certain younger disabled people, and those with kidney failure on dialysis for greater than three months.

A U.S. citizen who is at least 65 years old is eligible for Medicare if the person or the person's spouse worked for at least ten years in Medicare-covered employment. A person under 65 can get Medicare if the person is a dialysis or kidney-transplant patient or has received Social Security disability benefits for 24 months.

Medicare is divided into Part A (Hospital Insurance) and Part B (Medical Insurance). Part A helps pay for care in a hospital, skilled nursing facility, home health and hospice care. Part B helps pay for physicians, outpatient care, and various other services not covered in Part A.

Medicare Hospice Benefit

Medicare coverage for hospice care is available only if:

1. the patient is eligible for Medicare Part A;
2. the patient's physician and hospice Medical Director certify that the patient is terminally ill with a life expectancy of six months or less;
3. the patient signs a statement choosing hospice care instead of standard medical benefits for the terminal illness; and
4. the patient receives care from a Medicare-approved hospice program.

When all requirements are met, Medicare covers physician services, nursing care, medical equipment and supplies, outpatient drugs for symptom relief and pain management, home health aides, physical and occupational therapy, speech therapy, and dietary and other counseling.

Not covered are treatment for terminal illness except for symptom management and/or pain control, care provided by another hospice not arranged by the patient's hospice, and duplication of required hospice services by another provider.

Social Security Disability

A person can receive Social Security (SS) disability benefits at any age. To qualify, a person must have contributed to Social Security long enough and recently enough through their employment. In most cases, a person needs 20 credits earned in the last ten years ending in the year of becoming disabled. However, younger persons may qualify with fewer credits:

- <u>Before age 24</u> – Six credits earned in the three-year period ending when the disability began
- <u>Age 24–31</u> – Must have credit for working half the time between age 21 and the time of becoming disabled
- <u>Age 31 and up</u> – Varies depending on the age disabled

Disability is determined by a team consisting of an MD and a Disability Evaluation Specialist. Disability is determined in a step-by-step process involving five questions:

1. <u>Are you working?</u> – A person earning greater than $500/month cannot be determined as disabled.
2. <u>Is your condition severe?</u> – The impairment must interfere with basic work-related activities for the claim to be considered.
3. <u>Is the condition found in the list of disabling impairments?</u> – Social Security maintains a list of major body impairments sufficiently severe to warrant automatic determination of disability. If the condition is not on the list, Social Security will determine whether it is severe enough to warrant disability.
4. <u>Can the person do the same type of work previously performed?</u> – If the condition is severe, but not the same or of equal severity as an impairment on the list, then Social Security must determine if it interferes with the person's ability to do the work performed in the last 15 years. If it does not, the claim can be denied.
5. <u>Can you do any type of work?</u>

Note: A person must receive Social Security disability for 24 months to be eligible for Medicare.

Medicaid

Generally, Medicaid is awarded if a person is eligible for Supplemental Security Income (SSI). Medicaid covers health-care costs for persons who are blind, disabled, or fall below a certain percentile of the poverty level. Unlike Medicare, Medicaid offers a perscription benefit. Most patients in nursing homes are covered by Medicaid after depleting their personal funds.

Private Insurance

Different policies pay different amounts. In general, private insurance does not pay as well as state and federal programs except in the case of Railroad Retirement, Champus, and certain pensions. Supplemental policies are almost always necessary to cover all expenses.

The Medically Indigent
Example: Jefferson County, Alabama

- Covered in Jefferson County through the Jefferson Health System.
- The patient must be a Jefferson County resident.
- The patient is assessed according to income and the number of persons in the family.
- A scale based on the federal poverty guidelines is used to determine the amount of assistance given.

Access to Medical Care
at Life's End

Selected Readings

Economics of Palliative Care

Payne, S. K., P. Coyne, and T. J. Smith. "The Health Economics of Palliative Care." *Oncology* 16 (2002): 801–808.

Location of Death

Hansen, S. M., S. W. Tolle, and D. P. Martin. "Factors Associated with Lower Rates of In-hospital Death." *Journal of Palliative Medicine* 5 (2002): 677–685.

Access in a Diverse Society

Brenner, P. R. "Issues of Access in a Diverse Society." *The Hospice Journal* 12 (1997): 9–16.

Policy Recommendations

Sandy, L. G. "Homeostasis without Reserve—the Risk of Health System Collapse." *New England Journal of Medicine* 347 (2002): 1971–1975.

Von Gunten, C. F., F. D. Ferris, R. D'Antuono, and L. L. Emanuel. "Recommendations to Improve End-of-life Care through Regulatory Change in U.S. Health-care Financing." *Journal of Palliative Medicine* 5 (2002): 35–41.

2.2 Medicare Hospice Benefit

Key Points

1. Hospice care, now available in most communities in the United States, offers palliative medical care and serves patients and families as a unit with emotional, social, and spiritual support.

2. Patients certified as terminally ill with a life expectancy of less than six months may elect to receive hospice care.

3. A multidisciplinary team collaborates with patient and family to provide hospice care.

4. Hospice services include medical equipment and supplies, medication for pain and symptom control, chemotherapy and radiation (if for palliation), grief counseling, and bereavement support.

5. Hospice benefits cover hospital services for short-term symptom control and temporary respite care to relieve family caregivers. They do not cover curative treatments or extensive evaluations inconsistent with the hospice approach.

    Medicare continues to cover treatment for conditions other than the terminal illness.

6. Patients, initially certified for two 90-day periods, may be re-certified for an unlimited number of 60-day periods if the condition is still terminal with life expectancy within six months.

7. Discharge from hospice occurs if prognosis improves or if patient wishes to seek curative treatment. Patient may be readmitted if becomes eligible due to declining health.

Medicare Hospice Benefit

The Palliative Response

History of Hospice Benefit

- 1983—Federal Government adds hospice benefit to Medicare Part A

  National benefit for Medicare-eligible patients

  Developed by Center for Medicare and Medicaid Services (CMS) and Congress

  Following successful demonstration project
- Home hospice programs now available in most communities in USA

Support for Hospice Services

- Other sources

  Medicaid

  VA

  Private insurance

  Charity care by the hospice itself
- Accessibility

  All patients treated the same regardless of Medicare coverage

What Is Hospice Care?
Palliative Care

- Medical support
- Emotional support
- Social support
- Spiritual support

Whom Does Hospice Serve?

- People with terminal illness
- Family unit of patient

Settings of Hospice Services

- Home
- Nursing home
- Hospice facility
- Hospital

Medicare Hospice Eligibility Process

- Patient eligibility
  Medicare Part A (Hospital Insurance)
- Medical certification
  Terminal illness— < six months life expectancy
  Hospice medical director and patient's physician
- Patient election
  Patient elects hospice care over routine Medicare
- Program eligibility
  Medicare-approved hospice program

Prognostication Criteria

- Prognostication is often difficult
- Illness-specific criteria to support prognosis of less than six months

Certification requirement

- "Six-months rule" often discourages referral and shortens hospice time for eligible patients who could benefit from earlier referral
- No penalty for patient or physician if survival exceeds six months

Multidisciplinary Hospice Team

- Patient and family
- RNs, LPNs, Home health aides (nursing care)
- Social work
- Chaplain (pastoral care)
- Physician
- Trained volunteers
- Pysical/Occupational/Speech therapists, nutritionist

Types of Services Covered by Hospice

- Medical equipment and supplies
- Medication for pain and symptom control
- Professional services of multidisciplinary team
- Clinical services

Hospice Clinical Services

- Treatment that is palliative in nature (e.g., palliative chemotherapy and radiation)
- Counseling and bereavement services for family for up to one year after death

Hospital Services Covered by Hospice

- Symptom control
  Short-term inpatient care if symptoms not controlled at home
- Respite care
  Provides temporary relief to family or primary caregiver
  Up to five days

Types of Services Not Covered by Hospice

- Treatment to cure a terminal illness
- Extensive evaluations not consistent with hospice approach

  Focus is comfort, support, and symptom management

Medicare Coverage
Other Conditions

- Medicare continues to cover care and treatment for conditions other than the terminal illness

  Example: 66-year-old man with CRF on dialysis develops metastatic lung cancer
- Medicare hospice benefit covers admission to hospice for lung cancer
- Medicare A continues to cover dialysis

Co-Payments

- Medicare A and B

  80% of charges/ 20% co-payment
- Medicare hospice

  Medicare per diem reimbursement to hospice

  No co-pay for hospice

  May be a 5% co-pay for inpatient respite care
- Medications

  Patients responsible for medications not related to diagnosis

  May be a $5 co-pay for some prescriptions

Time Limit

- Certification

  Patient initially certified for two 90-day periods

  Certified thereafter for an unlimited number of 60-day periods
- Re-certification

  Medical director and physician review status

  Certify that prognosis is still terminal

  Certify that it is probable that the patient will die within the next six months

Hospice Discharge

- Patient becomes ineligible

  Remission

  Significant improvement

  No penalty for discharge

  Patient may be readmitted if becomes eligible due to declining health
- Patient elects discharge

  Some patients choose to be discharged to seek "curative" care not provided by hospice

Medicare Hospice Benefit
A Palliative Response

Hospice care is the ideal palliative response for many terminally ill patients and their families.

Refer early for maximum benefit.

Selected Readings

Overview of Hospice Care

Byock, I. R. "End-of-life Care: A Public Health Crisis and an Opportunity for Managed Care." *The American Journal of Managed Care* 7 (2001): 1123–1132.

Emanuel, E. J., A. Ash, W. Yu, G. Gazelle, N. G. Levinsky, O. Saynina, M. McClellan, and M. Moskositz. "Managed Care, Hospice Use, Site of Death, and Medical Expenditures in the Last Year of Life." *Archives of Internal Medicine* 162 (2002): 1722–1728.

Health Care Financing Administration. "Medicare Hospice Benefits: A Special Way of Caring for People Who Have a Terminal Illness." U.S. Department of Health and Human Services: Publication No. HCFA 02154, 2000.

Prognostication and Referral

Christakis, N. A. and E. B. Lamont. "Extent and Determinants of Error in Doctors' Prognoses in Terminally Ill Patients: Prospective Cohort Study." *British Medical Journal* 320 (2000): 469–473.

Friedman, B. T., M. K. Harwood, and M. Shields. "Barriers and Enablers to Hospice Referrals: An Expert Overview." *Journal of Palliative Medicine* 5 (2002): 73–84.

McCarthy, E. P., R. B. Burns, R. B. Davis, and R. S. Phillips. "Barriers to Hospice Care among Older Patients Dying with Lung and Colorectal Cancer." *Journal of Clinical Oncology* 21 (2003): 728–735.

Family Caregiver Burden

Andrews, S. C. "Caregiver Burden and Symptom Distress in People with Cancer Receiving Hospice Care." *Oncology Nursing Forum* 28 (2001): 1469–1474.

2.3 Nursing-Home Care

Key Points

1. Nursing-home care provides room and board; 24 hours/day assistance with Activities of Daily Living (ADL); and psychosocial, physical, and occupational therapies.

2. Factors leading to nursing home placement include inability to perform ADL, incontinence, functional impairment, cognitive impairment, and lack of social support system.

3. Medicare Part A covers care by a skilled nursing facility (SNF), hospice, or home health. Medicare reimbursement is 100% for 20 days ($100 co-pay for days 21–100).

4. Medicare Part B covers physician services, lab work, x-rays, and outpatient physical, occupational, and speech therapy (PT, OT, ST).

5. Medicaid, the payer of last resort, is a joint federal and state program that reimburses for custodial care (room and board) and medications for impoverished persons (income < $1500/month) in SNF.

6. Transfer summaries for admissions to SNF from hospital should include discharge diagnoses, most recent labs, procedures, study results, and Next of Kin (NOK)/Surrogate/Power of Attorney (POA).

7. Nursing-home orders should <u>avoid:</u>
   - PRN Orders—Medications should be scheduled
   - Open-ended orders—Use stop dates
   - Inappropriate PT/OT/ST consults—e.g., severe dementia
   - Restrictive Diets—#1 cause of weight loss in nursing homes
   - Patterned Blood Sugars
   - "Consult GI for PEG placement"—Understand the goals of the patient and family; it is not "nursing-home policy" to tube-feed patients who cannot take PO
   - Discharging with Foley Catheter, with certain exceptions

8. Ensure that each medication prescribed is indicated and has a corresponding diagnosis. Start low and go slow. Order as BID/TID etc., instead of qXhrs. Follow federal prescribing guidelines of Beer's List.

Nursing-Home Care

The Palliative Response

Levels of Long-Term Care

- Retirement communities
- Assisted living
- Skilled nursing facilities (SNF)

Nursing-Home Care

- 24 hr/day nursing care
- Assistance with Activities of Daily Living (ADL)
  Feeding, bathing, toileting, dressing
- Psychosocial, physical, occupational therapy
- Room and board

Factors Affecting Nursing-Home Placement

- Inability to perform ADL
  Incontinence is primary reason for nursing-home admission
- Functional impairment
- Cognitive impairment
- Lack of social support system

Medicare and Medicaid

Medicare Part A Coverage
- Skilled nursing facility
- Hospice
- Home health
- Dialysis
- 100% reimbursement for 20 days ($100 co-pay for days 21–100)

Medicare and Medicaid

Medicare Part B Coverage
- Physician services
- Lab
- X-ray
- "Outpatient" PT/OT/ST
- Must elect to pay in

Medicare and Medicaid
Medicaid Coverage

- Custodial care (room and board) in SNF
- Medications
- The payer of last resort
- Joint federal and state program
- Reimbursement varies from state to state

Medicaid Eligibility

- Impoverished (Income < $1500/ month)
- Spend-down to qualify
  Exemptions: automobile, life insurance, personal effects < $4000, real property in certain classes
- Look back 36 months for assets transferred as gifts, etc.
- Formula: Assets/Mo. NH Cost = Period Ineligible

Admissions to SNF

- From home
- From hospital with transfer summary
  D/C diagnoses
  Most recent labs
  Procedures
  Results studies
  NOK/Surrogate/POA
  Code status
  Candidate for rehab? If no, why not?
    - *Goals*
    - *Potential*

Skilled Nursing Facility
Skills of Care Available

- Feeding tubes
- Fractures
- IVs, IMs
- Ostomy care
- Wound care
- Physical therapy
- Occupational therapy
- Speech therapy

Orders to Avoid

- PRNs
  If a medication is needed, it should be scheduled (e.g., analgesics)
- Open-ended orders
  Use stop dates (e.g., antibiotics, opthalmic preparations, dermatologic preparations)
- Inappropriate PT/OT/ST consults
  (e.g., Severe dementia—unable to learn, recall)

Avoid Restrictive Diets

- #1 cause of weight loss in NH
- Have no place in NH setting; residents should be able to eat anything they can
- Remember to specify consistency
- Request "spoonfeed" or "assist with feeding"
- Exception—short-stay rehab for otherwise functional patient

Avoid Patterned Blood Sugars

- In stable Type 2s
- If unstable for finite period (three days, one week) with insulin titration per nursing-home physician

Avoid "Consult GI for PEG Placement"

- Understand the goals of the patient and family
- It is not "nursing-home policy" to tube-feed patients who cannot take PO

Avoid Discharging with Foley Catheter

Exceptions
- For wound healing
  "d/c Foley when wound healed"
- Hip, LE fracture
  "d/c Foley when fracture healed"
- Neurogenic bladder

Prescribing Drugs in NH

- Ensure it is indicated
  Each drug prescribed needs a corresponding diagnosis
- "Start low and go slow"
- Prescribe low-cost equivalents when possible
- Order as BID/TID, etc., instead of qXhrs

The Beer's List

- Delineates prescribing practices in NH
- Adopted as federal guideline on prescribing
- Used by state surveyors in evaluating drug prescribing in NH
- Does not prohibit the prescribing of drugs but requires physician documentation on the use of certain drugs, effectively proscribing their use

Examples of Beer's List

Drug	Strength	Dosing Schedule
FeSO4	325mg QD	GI side effects, limited indications (blood loss)
Dig	0.0125mg QD	Renal impairment, risk of toxicity
Propoxiphene	Don't prescribe	Limited efficacy, toxic metabolites in renal insufficiency
Benzodiazepine	Any	Don't prescribe unless willing to give a legitimate psychiatric diagnosis
Tricyclics	Any	Don't prescribe unless there is no other drug for sleep, neuropathy, or depression
Antipsychotic	Any	Don't prescribe unless documented psychiatric diagnosis, dementia w/agitation, hospice (N/V)

Nursing-Home Care

Selected Readings

Overview of Nursing Home Care at Life's End

Cartwright, J. C. "Nursing Homes and Assisted-Living Facilities as Places for Dying." *Annual Review of Nursing Research* 20 (2002): 231–264.

Hanson, L. C., M. Henderson, and M. Menon. "As Individual as Death Itself: A Focus Group Study of Terminal Care in Nursing Homes." *Journal of Palliative Care* 5 (2002): 117–125.

Miller, S. C. and V. Mor. "The Role of Hospice Care in the Nursing Home Setting." *Journal of Palliative Care* 5 (2002): 271–277.

Parker-Oliver, D. "Hospice Experience and Perceptions in Nursing Homes." *Journal of Palliative Medicine* 5 (2002): 713–720.

Hospice Care in Assisted-Living Communities

Dixon, S., J. Fortner, and S. S. Travis. "Barriers, Challenges, and Opportunities Related to the Provision of Hospice Care in Assisted-Living Communities." *American Journal of Hospice and Palliative Care* 19 (2002): 187–192.

Educating Long-Term Care Facilities in End-of-Life Care

Steel, K., M. Ribbe, J. Ahronheim, H. Hedrick, P. A. Selwyn, W. Forman, and T. Keay. "Incorporating Education on Palliative Care into the Long-Term Care Setting." *Journal of the American Geriatrics Society* 47 (1999): 904–907.

Withholding or Withdrawing Artificial Nutrition and Hydration

Onwuteaka-Phillipsen, B. D., H. R. Pasman, A. Kruit, A. van der Heide, M. W. Ribbe, and G. van der Wal. "Withholding or Withdrawing Artificial Administration of Food and Fluids in Nursing-Home Patients." *Age and Ageing* 30 (2001): 459–465.

—— Comment in *Age and Ageing* 2001: 436–438.

Physician-Assisted Suicide in the Frail Elderly

Smith, W. B. "Physician-Assisted Suicide and Euthanasia's Impact on the Frail Elderly: Autonomy or a License to Kill? Some Ethical Perspectives." *Journal of Long-Term Home Health Care* 17 (1998): 42–49.

2.4 Ethical Considerations

Key Points

1. The primary ethical principles in Palliative Care are autonomy, beneficence, non-maleficence, justice, and informed consent.

2. Ethical principles can sometimes conflict with each other.
   Unlimited or unguided patient autonomy can conflict with beneficence, non-maleficence and justice.

3. An action is ethical if its intent is beneficent even if outcome is negative.
   Double effect is the recognition that any action taken on behalf of the patient can have multiple impacts, both positive and negative. Thus, if taken to its logical conclusion, the principle "First of All, Do No Harm" would paralyze physicians.

4. Use of opioid medications for relief of pain or dyspnea is accepted and expected as standard pain and symptom management.
   The medical system too often under treats pain; providers have recently faced criminal prosecution for under treatment of pain in terminally ill patients.

5. Forgoing life-sustaining treatment applies to a number of interventions beyond ventilator support.
   The decision to withdraw or not begin a therapy includes such interventions as CPR, dialysis, tube feeding and medications as well as ventilator support.

6. The purpose of intentional/terminal sedation is symptom-relief, not death (double effect).
   Intentional sedation seeks to provide relief from severe, unrelenting physical symptoms that are irreversible and unresponsive to maximal symptom control.

Ethical Considerations

The Palliative Response

The Ethical Principle of Autonomy

Patient Choice

Self-determination in decisions regarding accepting or refusing specific treatment.

The Ethical Principle of Beneficence

Do Good

Working out together what would be in the best interest of a patient.

The Ethical Principle of Non-Maleficence

Minimize Harm

Protection of patients from injury and iatrogenic harm.

Includes wise counseling as a component of informed consent.

The Ethical Principle of Justice

Fair use of available resources for health care

Conflict of Autonomy with Other Principles

- In the recent history of medicine, autonomy often has been considered the most important of the ethical principles

- Unlimited or unguided patient autonomy can conflict with the ethical principles of beneficence, nonmaleficence, and justice

The Ethical Principle of Informed Consent

Voluntary and informed agreement to specific treatment or plan of care

Capacity

The presence of sufficient mental capacity to exercise autonomy and to give consent

Beneficence and Double Effect

- Any action taken on the behalf of a patient has potential for multiple impacts, positive and negative, on a patient's well-being

- An action is ethical if its intent is beneficent even if a negative outcome should occur

Limiting Considerations
First of All, Do No Harm

If carried to its logical conclusion, this principle would prevent physicians from participating in any patient-care decisions; since any action, however harmless it may appear, could have negative consequences for an individual patient

Exercise in Ethical Decision-Making

Six different scenarios will be described regarding care at Life's End. As a group you will fill out a table regarding:
- Certainty of death
- Requirement for patient competence
- Physician involvement in the interventions
- Legal status of the intervention
- Ethical consensus

Interventions
Standard Pain Management

- Use of opioid medications for the relief of pain or dyspnea is accepted and expected
- Intent is control of pain or other symptoms
- Medical system too often under-treats pain
- Some providers have faced criminal actions for inadequate pain control for terminally ill patients

Foregoing Life-Sustaining Therapy

- Discussions often limited to ventilator support
- Includes a number of interventions beyond ventilator support

  CPR

  Dialysis

  Tube feeding

  Medications

- Includes withdrawing a therapy or making a proactive decision not to begin a treatment

Voluntary Cessation of Eating and Drinking

- A rare event requiring sustained will power
- Some may consider this suicide
- Evaluation of depression and capacity are appropriate

Intentional/Terminal Sedation

- May be indicated for severe unrelenting physical pain or other distressing symptoms, such as delirium or dyspnea, which are not reversible and not responding to maximal symptom control
- Patient is sedated—usually with a combination of opioids, benzodiazepines and haloperidol—because sleeping provides respite from the symptoms
- Purpose of the treatment is relief of symptoms, not death (double effect)

Physician-Assisted Suicide
Oregon Regulations

Physician provides the means for patient to take his/her own life

- Patient must make request in writing
- Waiting period
- Second physician must certify illness as terminal
- May be a psychiatric evaluation
- Patient fills prescription for barbiturate to use at his/her discretion
- Patient must take the medication unaided by staff or family

Voluntary Active Euthanasia

Physician, upon patient request, administers lethal medication by injection or oral route

- Patient must be competent
- Illegal and likely to be prosecuted
- Limited and controversial support for this practice

The Ethical Principle of Beneficence

Do Good

While all the ethical principles are important, working with the patient/family toward beneficence often, in the end, will achieve the other principles.

Intervention	Certainty of Death	Patient Competence	Physician Involvement	Legal Status	Ethical Consensus
Standard pain management					
Foregoing life-sustaining therapy					
Voluntarily stopping eating and drinking					
Terminal sedation: heavy sedation to escape pain, shortness of breath, other severe symptoms					
Physician-assisted suicide					
Voluntary active euthanasia					

Ethical Considerations

Selected Readings

Emerging Ethical Issues in Palliative Care

Burt, R. A. "The Supreme Court Speaks: Not Assisted Suicide but a Constitutional Right to Palliative Care." *New England Journal of Medicine* 337 (1997): 1234–1236.

Pellegrino, E. D. "Emerging Ethical Issues in Palliative Care." *Journal of the American Medical Association* 279 (1998): 1521–1522.

Quill, T. E., B. C. Lee, and S. Nunn. "Palliative Treatments of Last Resort: Choosing the Least Harmful Alternative." *Annals of Internal Medicine* 132 (2000): 488–493.

The Medical Futility Debate

Burt, R. A. "The Medical Futility Debate: Patient Choice, Physician Obligation, and End-of-life Care." *Journal of Palliative Medicine* 5 (2002): 249–254.

Ditillo, B. A. "Should There Be a Choice for Cardiopulmonary Resuscitation when Death Is Expected? Revisiting an Old Idea whose Time Is Yet to Come." *Journal of Palliative Medicine* 5 (2002): 107–116.

Gazelle, G. "The Slow Code—Should Anyone Rush to Its Defense?" *New England Journal of Medicine* 338 (1998): 467–469.

Krieger, B. P. "Futile Ventilator Support: Clinical and Ethical Aspects of Withdrawal." *The Journal of Critical Illness* 15 (2000): 483–493.

Lo, B., L. Dornbrand, L. E. Wolf, and M. Groman. "The Wendland Case—Withdrawing Life Support from Incompetent Patients who Are not Terminally Ill." *New England Journal of Medicine* 346 (2002): 1489–1493.

Virtue Ethics

Giblin, M. J. "Beyond Principles: Virtue Ethics in Hospice and Palliative Care." *American Journal of Hospice and Palliative Care* 19 (2002): 235–239.

McDonagh, J. and V. Ljungkvist. "Learning Empathy: Medical School and the Care of the Dying Patient." *Journal of Palliative Medicine* 2 (1999): 383–389.

2.5 Physician–Assisted Suicide

Key Points

1. Physician-assisted suicide (PAS) is legal only in Oregon.
   PROCEDURE: Applicants must be Oregon residents whom two physicians certify as terminally ill with a prognosis of less than six months. Applicant must request PAS in writing and undergo a waiting period during which a psychiatric evaluation may be requested. Patient receives barbiturate prescription that he must take <u>unaided</u> when and if he decides to do so.

2. Patients requesting PAS are usually attempting to control social and emotional, rather than physical, suffering.
   Palliative care can manage most physical suffering. Motivation for requesting PAS includes fear of dependency, lack of ability to care for self, and becoming a burden on others.

3. Respond to request for PAS by assessing effectiveness of palliative care and revising care plan to address patient concerns.
   Reevaluate patient's response to interventions, including treatment for depression over the course of the illness; PAS requests are usually not persistent over time.

4. Be open to discussing PAS with patients. Maintain therapeutic relationship with patient despite disagreement with PAS.
   Listen to patient's concerns, remain professional and calm and normalize patient's thoughts about PAS. Don't freak out! Continue to support patient and family and to seek other sources of support. Continue to reduce and relieve suffering at Life's End. Neither abandon nor judge the patient.

5. Prepare for patient-clinician interactions by developing expertise in dealing with dying.
   Expertise in dealing with the dying process includes ability to control symptoms, manage the entire course of terminal illness, handle emergencies or expected complications, and access community resources and the assistance of interdisciplinary team.

6. Intentional sedation, sometimes the only means of providing relief from intolerable suffering not controlled by aggressive symptom management, is <u>not</u> PAS or euthanasia. Its intention is the relief of suffering. The intention of PAS is the death of the patient.

Physician–Assisted Suicide

The Palliative Response

Physician-Assisted Suicide
Legal Only in Oregon

Eligibility
- Patient must be Oregon resident
- Two physicians must certify illness as terminal with prognosis of less than six months

---

Physician-Assisted Suicide

Initial procedure
- Must request PAS in writing
- Waiting period
- Psychiatric evaluation may be requested

PAS procedure
- Patient receives barbiturate prescription
- Patient decides when/if to use medication
- Patient must take medication unaided

The Experience in Oregon

Requests and use
- 50–75 patients per year formally request PAS
- About one third of those who obtain medication actually use it for PAS

The palliative alternative
- Oregon has a high utilization rate for hospice and palliative-care services—partially in response to the debate and the Death with Dignity Law

---

National Survey Data
PAS

Terminally-ill patients (988)
- 60% support PAS in hypothetical situations
- 10% had seriously considered PAS in their own situations

Primary-care physicians
- About 25% reported a request for PAS

Oncologists
- About 50% reported a request for PAS

Characteristics of Patients
Requesting PAS

- Anyone might think about PAS and hastened death in the context of a serious and life-threatening illness
- Those requesting PAS are more likely:
  Male
  White
  Higher level of education attainment
  Higher socioeconomic class
  Not active in a religious practice

Reasons for Seeking PAS

Emotional and social suffering
- Control
  Over the situation and terminal illness
- Fear
  Dependency
  Lack of ability to care for self

  Becoming a burden on others

Responding to Request
Attitudinal Guidelines

Be open to discuss PAS
- Listen to patient's concerns
- Remain professional and calm
- Normalize patient's thoughts about PAS

  Don't Freak Out

When a Patient Asks about PAS

Clarify
- Patients commonly use unclear language secondary to concern about physician's response to request
- Ask in calm, supportive way for clarification about what assistance patient is seeking

When a Patient Asks about PAS

Explore reasons for request
- Fear of uncontrolled symptoms
- Fear of loss of "dignity" or control
- Burden on family
- Each patient may have unique reasons

When a Patient Asks about PAS

Assess effectiveness of palliative-care interventions
- Physical symptoms
- Social support
- Spiritual concerns
- Emotional aspects (especially depression)

When a Patient Asks about PAS

Revise the care plan
- Address and respond to patient concerns
- Reevaluate response to interventions over the course of the illness
  PAS requests are usually not persistent over time

Palliative Response to the Underlying Suffering

In response to a request for PAS:
- Assess and manage untreated depression
- Manage physical suffering
  Most can be managed such that patients have the capacity to bare the distress

Response to PAS Request
Summary

- Physician-assisted suicide is illegal and not condoned as an ethical practice
- Make explicit that physician-assisted suicide is not a clinical option
  but
- Reassure patient and family that you and the interdisciplinary team will support them throughout the dying process

Response to PAS Request
Summary

Maintain therapeutic relationship
- Despite disagreement about PAS
- Continue to be a source of support and care for patient and family
- Neither abandon nor judge
- Continue to seek sources of support
- Continue to reduce and relieve suffering at Life's End

Preparation for Managing PAS Request

Expertise in dealing with dying process is the best preparation
- Expertise in symptom control
- Knowledge about the time course of illness
- Preparation for emergencies or expected complications
- Knowledge about community resources
- Ease in working with interdisciplinary team

Uncontrollable Symptoms
The Palliative Response

- Admission
  Inpatient palliative care or hospice unit
- Consultation
- Multidisciplinary care
  To manage symptoms across a broad spectrum of suffering

Uncontrollable Symptoms
The Palliative Response

Intentional sedation
- When aggressive symptom management does not control symptoms
- When only means of relieving distressing symptom is sedation to a sleeplike state
- Intention is relief from intolerable suffering
  Intention is not death
  Not considered PAS or euthanasia, in which intention is the death of the patient

Physician-Assisted Suicide

Selected Readings

Overview of Issue

Quill, T. E., D. E. Meier, S. D. Block, and J. A. Billings. "The Debate over Physician-Assisted Suicide: Empirical Data and Convergent Views." *Annals of Internal Medicine* 128 (1998): 552–558.

Sachs, G. A., J. C. Ahronheim, J. A. Rhymes, L. Volicer, and J. Lynn. "Good Care of Dying Patients: The Alternative to Physician-Assisted Suicide and Euthanasia." *Journal of the American Geriatrics Society* 43 (1995): 553–562.

Snyder, L. and D. Sulmasy. "Physician-Assisted Suicide." *Annals of Internal Medicine* 135 (2001): 209–216.

Physician-Patient Interactions

Back, A. L., H. Starks, C. Hsu, J. R. Gordon, A. Bharucha, and R. A. Pearlman. "Clinician-Patient Interactions about Requests for Physician-Assisted Suicide." *Archives of Internal Medicine* 162 (2002): 1257–1265.

Smith, W. B. "Physician-Assisted Suicide and Euthanasia's Impact on the Frail Elderly: Autonomy or a License to Kill? Some Ethical Perspectives." *Journal of Long Term Home Health Care* 17 (1998): 42–49.

The Oregon Experience

Ganzini, L., H. D. Nelson, M. A. Lee, D. F. Kraemer, T. A. Scdhmidt, and M. A. Delorit. "Oregon Physicians' Attitudes about and Experiences with End-of-life Care since Passage of the Oregon Death with Dignity Act." *Journal of the American Medical Association* 285 (2001): 2363–2369.

Ganzini, L., H. D. Nelson, T. A. Schmidt, D. F. Kraemer, M. A. Delorit, and M. A. Lee. "Physicians' Experiences with the Oregon Death with Dignity Act." *New England Journal of Medicine* 342 (2000): 557–563.

The Netherlands' Experience

Groenewoud, J. H., A. van der Heide, B. D. Onwuteaka-Philipsen, D. L. Willems, P. J. van der Maas, and G. van der Wal. "Clinical Problems with the Performance of Euthanasia and Physician-Assisted Suicide in the Netherlands." *New England Journal of Medicine* 342 (2000): 551–556.

Attitudes of Terminally-Ill Patients and Their Caregivers

Emanuel, E. J., D. L. Fairclough, and L. L. Emanuel. "Attitudes and Desires Related to Euthanasia and Physician-Assisted Suicide among Terminally-Ill Patients and Their Givers." *Journal of the American Medical Association* 284 (2000): 2460–2468.

Emotional Suffering: The Palliative Response

3.1 Delirium

Key Points

1. Delirium is deadly.

   When people become delirious, they stop eating, drinking fluids, and taking medicines. They may injure themselves or be placed in restraints. The prognosis is grave if the delirium does not clear. The delirium complicates and interferes with treatment of other aspects of the illness and often results in the use of restraints.

2. Delirium is common.

   15–20% of people who are hospitalized may experience delirium, and 80–90% may have some delirium in the days and weeks before death.

3. Delirium causes extreme emotional suffering.

   A delirious individual is often frightened, agitated, and upset. Most important, the delirium interferes with meaningful personal interactions with family, friends, and professional staff at Life's End.

4. Delirium is treatable and in some cases reversible.

   The physician must individualize the treatment of delirium to maximize the patient's comfort and safety. The physician must temper the search for etiology and any corrective efforts with consideration of the burden of treatment on individuals at Life's End. In any case, treatment of the symptoms with neuroleptics (haloperidol) is usually appropriate.

5. Mistreatment with benzodiazepines (lorazepam) often exacerbates delirium.

   Health-care providers often misinterpret the agitation associated with delirium as anxiety and fear. Treatment with benzodiazepines (lorazepam) for agitation may lead to a vicious cycle of escalating doses that exacerbates the underlying delirium.

Delirium

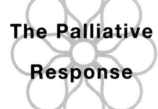

The Palliative Response

A Definition

- Confusion
- Sudden onset
- Waxing and waning
- Disturbed level of consciousness
- Labile emotions
- Delusions
- Disorientation
- Hallucinations (usually visual)
- Altered sleep/ wake cycle
- Psycho-motor agitation or somnolence
- Decreased cognitive function

Delirium Is Deadly

Delirious patients
- Stop eating
- Stop drinking fluids
- Stop taking important medications
- May fall and injure themselves
- Often are placed in restraints and suffer complications such as aspiration and decubitus
- Interferes with assessment and treatment of other symptoms

Delirium Is Deadly

Delirious patients have a grave prognosis
- The delirium may herald the last days of life in a hospice patient with irreversible illness
- In the last days of life, the treatment may concentrate on the control of the symptoms rather than correction of the underlying cause

Delirium Is Deadly

- Failure to recognize and adequately treat delirium in patients who do not have life-limiting illnesses greatly increases their morbidity and mortality

Delirium Is Common

- 80% of people experience some delirium during the final week of life
- 15–20% admitted to hospitals with cancer experience some delirium

Delirium Causes Extreme Emotional Suffering

- Causes a person to be frightened, agitated, and upset
- Increases the use of restraints

Delirium Causes Extreme Emotional Suffering

Most important, delirium at Life's End interferes with meaningful communication and interaction:

with family and friends

with professional staff (physician, nurses, clergy, counselors)

Management of Delirium

Symptomatic and supportive therapies

Indicated when the burden of evaluation and treatment of the underlying causes of the delirium outweighs the benefits.

Management of Delirium

Considerations

- Work-up of delirium may be limited by the home and hospice setting
- Causes of delirium are often multifactorial
- When a distinct cause is found, it often is irreversible

Management of Delirium

- The comfort of the person suffering from delirium is paramount
- Symptomatic treatment can begin with or without a diagnostic work-up
- Good clinical judgment determines the extent to which to look for and pursue reversible causes of delirium

Management of Delirium
Medications

*benzodiazepines   opioids
anticholinergics antiemetics steroids*

- It is important to simplify the regimen
- It is important to stop unnecessary medications
- It is inappropriate to stop opioids if necessary to control pain and dyspnea
- It may be more reasonable to treat the delirium and continue the medication

Management of Delirium
Differential Diagnosis

- Electrolyte disturbances
- Hypercalcemia
- Hyper/Hypoglycemia
- Hyponatremia
- Uremia
- Hepatic encephalopathy
- Hypoxia

Management of Delirium
Differential Diagnosis

- Infections
  Pneumonia
  UTI
- CNS
  Metastatic spread of tumor
  Seizures
  Stroke or bleed
- Impaction/Constipation
- Urinary Retention

Management of Delirium

Agitation

Treatment with benzodiazepines (Ativan) for agitation associated with delirium may lead to a vicious cycle of escalating doses that only worsens the underlying delirium.

Evaluation of Delirium

- Relevant history
  New medications
  Known metastatic disease
- Physical exam
- Simple blood test
- More extensive work-up (CT scans, X-rays)
  May be warranted but physician must make the decision in light of the overall situation and course of the illness.

Treatment of Delirium
Specific Reversible Causes

- Fluids for dehydration
  IV, PO, SC
- Antibiotics
- Oxygen
- Lactulose
- Bladder catheterization
- Disimpaction

Treatment of Delirium
Fluids for Dehydration

- Caution must be used in using IV fluids
- Placement of IV line and restraints to protect the access may traumatize patient
- Fluid overload with edema and pulmonary congestion can add to suffering at Llife's End
- Use of fluids indicates a cautious, time-limited trial of therapy

Symptomatic Therapy
Neuroleptics

Haloperidol (Haldol) PO, IV, SC
- 0.5–1mg q2–12 hours
- May need to use multiple dose at first to control severe agitation

Chlorpromazine (Thorazine) PO, IV, IM
- 12.5–50mg q4–12 hours
- Use when more sedation is desirable
- Cannot be given SC

Symptomatic Therapy
Neuroleptics

Risperidone (Risperdal)
- 1–3mg PO q12 hours
- Popular because of reports of fewer side effects
- Only comes PO
- Costs $150–$250 for one-month supply

Symptomatic Therapy
Environmental

- Well-lighted room
- Quiet, calm, and familiar surroundings
- Presence of family or staff may be calming
- Restraints, IV lines, oxygen, and other instrumentation may contribute to agitation and suffering

Symptomatic Therapy
Benzodiazepines

Lorazepam (Ativan) PO,IV, SC
- 0.5–2mg q1–4 hours
- Sedation with the addition of a benzodiazepine may be appropriate if symptoms cannot be controlled and the delirium is causing suffering when death is imminent

Delirium
Palliative Care

Palliative-care consultation may be helpful with delirium at Life's End

- Reaching correct diagnosis
- Evaluation
- Treatment

Delirium
The Palliative Response

Delirium is common.
Delirium is deadly.
Comfort is paramount.

Delirium

Selected Readings

Prevalence of Delirium at Life's End

Nowels, D. E., C. Bublitz, C. T. Kassner, and J. S. Kutner. "Estimation of Confusion Prevalence in Hospice Patients." *Journal of Palliative Medicine* 5 (2002): 687–695.

Diagnosis and Management of Delirium at Life's End

Casarett, D. J. and S. K. Inouye. American College of Physicians—American Society of Internal Medicine End-of-Life Care Consensus Panel: "Diagnosis and Management of Delirium Near the End of Life." *Annals of Internal Medicine* 135 (2001): 32–40. Comments in: 137 (2002); discussion 295.

Ross, D. D. and C. S. Alexander. "Management of Common Symptoms in Terminally Ill Patients. Part II: Constipation, Delirium and Dyspnea." [Review] [39 refs]. *American Family Physician* 15; 64 (2001): 1019–1026.

Shuster, J. L. "Delirium, Confusion, and Agitation at the End of Life." *Journal of Palliative Medicine* 1 (1998): 177–186.

3.2 Anxiety

Key Points

1. Anxiety is an excessive state of apprehension that can contribute to suffering at Life's End by interfering with activities that give life meaning and purpose.

   Anxiety and fear are not the same thing. Fear may be appropriate, adaptive and protective. Anxiety is destructive. It can be continuous and ongoing, of incapacitating intensity, without a clear cause (autonomous), and can result in behavioral changes. Do not dismiss clinical anxiety as "normal" or acceptable.

2. Maintain high index of suspicion for anxiety, especially if behavioral changes manifest. Assess by routinely asking people if they are feeling fearful or anxious.

3. Seek to provide maximum resolution for anxiety.
   • Look for underlying causes;
   • Treat other symptoms aggressively;
   • Stop unnecessary medications and treatment;
   • Educate patient and family about treatment plan;
   • Reassure that some feelings of fear or uncertainty at Life's End may be normal but should be treated if too severe, continuous, or distressing.

4. Differential diagnosis is important in reaching diagnosis of anxiety.
   • Evaluate for pain, delirium, dyspnea, or other physical complication.
   • Consider medication side effect, pre-existing anxiety disorder, withdrawal state, and distress whose source is social, financial, spiritual, or existential.

5. Assess and treat or palliate the source of anxiety.
   • Consider pre-existent and pre-morbid depression and anxiety, Post-Traumatic Stress Disorder (PTSD), and death anxiety.
   • Re-assess control of symptoms, psycho-social-spiritual support, and medication regimen.

6. Medication is often helpful and appropriate in addressing anxiety at Life's End.

   Lorazepam (0.5–2mg q6–8 hours titrated as needed) is the most effective and commonly used medication. Behavioral and relaxation techniques are helpful in a small subset of people.

Anxiety

The Palliative Response

Anxiety versus Fear

Anxiety and fear are not the same.

Fear

- May be appropriate and adaptive
- Can be protective

Anxiety

Anxiety contributes to suffering at Life's End.

- State of apprehension, worry, uneasiness
- May arise from unknown internal source
- May be excessive/overwhelming response to external source
- Can be destructive

Signs of Distressing Anxiety

- Tension, restlessness
- Social withdrawal
- Avoidance
- Substance use and self-medication
- Rumination and dread
- Decreased capacity to cope

Anxiety at Life's End

- Prevalence is not clearly defined
- Often trivialized or dismissed
- Often is expected and accepted as inevitable
- Limits participation in planning for Goals of Care and for "living life"

Secondary Suffering

- Insomnia
- Depression
- GI upset
- Dysphagia
- Fatigue
- Withdrawal from social supports

Indications for Intervention

- Incapacitating intensity
  Anxiety exceeds capacity to bear suffering
- Behavioral changes
  Interferes with activities that give life meaning
- Continuous and ongoing

Assess Frequently

- Maintain high index of suspicion about anxiety
- Routinely ask patients if they are fearful or anxious
- Assess for causes when there are behavioral changes

Assess Cause

Physical
- Control of pain, dyspnea, other physical symptoms

Emotional
- Consider pre-existent depression and anxiety disorders
- Post-Traumatic Stress Disorder (PTSD)
- Assess emotional support

Assess Cause

Social and Spiritual
- Reassess support in community
- Contact pastoral care
- Contact Social Work services
- May need respite care or transfer to another venue of care if support is lacking and cannot be provided

Death Anxiety

- "Everyone wants to go to heaven, but no one wants to die to get there."

  —H. L. Mencken

- "I don't mind dying; I just don't want to be there when it happens."

  —Woody Allen

Differential Diagnosis

- Pain
- Delirium
- Fear
- Dyspnea
- Other physical complication
- Side effects of common medications
- Pre-existing anxiety disorder
- Withdrawl state
- Existential distress
- Social distress
- Financial distress
- Spiritual distress
- Coping style (type A)

Medications That May Contribute to Anxiety

- Theophylines
- Caffeine
- Albuterol
- Akathisia from antiemetics
- Withdrawal from opioids, benzodiazepine, or other substances

Medical Treatment

Medication is often helpful for anxiety at Life's End

- Lorazepam
  The most commonly used and effective
  0.5–2mg q6–8 hours titrated as needed
- Buspar probably not a good choice for immediate relief
- Xanax may have too short a half-life

Anxiety at Life's End
The Palliative Response

- Address patient's concerns to allay fears and reduce anxiety
- Evaluate other causes
- Treat other symptoms aggressively
- Stop unnecessary medications/ treatments
- Educate patient and family
  Anxiety at Life's End is common
  Treatment plan
  Solicit support and care
- Add medical treatment as necessary

Indications for Consultation

- PTSD
- Pre-existing anxiety disorder
- Anxiety not responding to management
- Consultation resources
  Palliative care
  Psychiatry

Anxiety at Life's End

Anxiety contributes to suffering and interferes with important personal work at Life's End.

Anxiety

Selected Readings

Barraclough, J. "ABC of Palliative Care. Depression, Anxiety, and Confusion [Review] [10 refs]. *British Medical Journal* 315 (1997): 1365–1368.

—— Comment: "A Comparative Study of Death Anxiety in Hospice and Emergency Nurses." In: *Journal of Advanced Nursing* 35 (2001): 384–385. 28 (1998): 700–706.

Hinshaw, D. B., J. M. Carnahan, and D. L. Johnson. "Depression, Anxiety and Asthenia in Advanced Illness." *Journal of the American College of Surgeons* 195 (2002): 271–277.

Paice, J. A. "Managing Psychological Conditions in Palliative Care." *American Journal of Nursing* 102 (2002): 36–42.

3.3 Depression

Key Points

1. Depression is common at Life's End.

   While depression is common, it is not universal at Life's End. Sadness is common but, unlike depression, sadness is not overwhelming, continuous, and pervasive. If the sadness a patient experiences is interfering with other important activities, it is probably depression.

2. Depression is often best diagnosed by asking people if they are depressed.

   Somatic symptoms like fatigue, appetite, and change in sleeping patterns cannot be used to diagnosis depression because they are present from other physical causes. Asking people directly to report if they are depressed is the most effective screening tool.

3. Anhedonia often accompanies depression.

   Anhedonia is the inability to experience pleasure. Even people at Life's End should be able to identify things, like family or friends, which still bring pleasure to their lives.

4. Uncontrolled physical and social suffering worsens depression.

   Good control of physical symptoms, especially pain and dyspnea, and social support in the residential setting at Life's End may help relieve depression.

5. Depression may respond to treatments like Selective Serotonin Reuptake Inhibitor (SSRI) and psychotherapy in the last months of life.

   Patients who have a better functional status may respond to SSRI in the last few months of life.

6. Depression may respond to treatment with psycho-stimulants in the last weeks or days of life.

   Methylphendalate (Ritalin) may be effective in treating depression within a few days of starting the medication. This might be helpful in the last few days of life or while waiting for an SSRI to work.

Depression

The Palliative Response

Depression Is Common at Life's End

- Clinical depression is never "appropriate"
- Some surveys report depression in up to 50% of palliative care patients
- Unrecognized and untreated depression causes substantial suffering at Life's End

Depression Can Be Diagnosed at Life's End

- Patients are often able to self-report if they are depressed
- Asking a patient "Are you depressed?" is a good screening test for depression
- Persons who say they are depressed probably are

Somatic Symptoms

Somatic symptoms are poor indicators of clinical depression because they can almost always have other causes.

- Fatigue
- Weakness
- Change in sleep patterns
- Change or decrease appetite and weight loss
- Constipation

Anhedonia
Marker for Depression

Anhedonia
(inability to experience pleasure)
- Can be a marker for depression regardless of whether the patient self-reports depression
- A patient who cannot stand the sight of grandchildren, previously the light of his/her life, is depressed

Suicide and Assisted Suicide

Requests for assisted dying
- Depression is a factor in requests for assisted dying

Suicide assessment and prevention
- "Have you thought of suicide?"
- "Do you have a plan?"
- "Will you contract with me that you will not kill yourself?"

Addressing Depression

Increase the capacity to bear suffering

- Good pain and symptom control

  Uncontrolled pain or other symptoms contribute greatly to depression

- Assist to maintain independence and Activities of Daily Life

- Social support

  Home hospice

  Encourage increased contact to maintain ties

Treating Depression
Antidepressants

Serotonin re-uptake inhibitors

- A mainstay for treatment of depression in palliative care
- Be aware of side effects such as anorexia
- Use in patients whose prognosis offers time for the treatment to be effective (2 to 6 months and functional status)

New atypical antidepressant holds promise

Treating Depression
Psychotherapy

- Formal psychotherapy is not commonly used in the palliative care/hospice setting
- Supportive counseling, listening, and attending to concerns can help support patients and families and increase the capacity to bear suffering
- Psychotherapy may be more directive and focused on problem-solving

Treating Depression
Psychostimulants

- Sometimes helpful in the last few weeks or days of life when depression is a major contributor to suffering
- If effective, will usually help within a few days rather than weeks-to-months
- May be helpful in conjunction with SSRI to treat symptoms quickly while awaiting the effect of the SSRI

Psychostimulants
Methylphendalate (Ritalin)

- Begin with 2.5–5mg at breakfast and lunch
- Titrate to effective dose at 5–15mg am and lunch
- Observe for adverse effects

  Anxiety

  Insomnia

  Agitation

Depression
The Palliative Response

Unrecognized and untreated depression causes substantial suffering at Life's End.

Screen for it.
Recognize it.
Treat it.

Clinical depression is never "appropriate."

Depression

Selected Readings

Overview

Barraclough, J. "ABC of Palliative Care: Depression, Anxiety, and Confusion." *British Medical Journal* 315 (1997): 1365–1368.

Massie, M. J. and D. K. Payne. "Depression and Anxiety." In: *Principles and Practice of Supportive Oncology* edited by A. M. Berger, R. K. Portenoy, and D. E. Weissman. New York: Lipincott Williams & Wilkins Healthcare, 3 (2000): 1–11.

Screening for Depression

Lloyd-Williams, M. "Is It Appropriate to Screen Palliative Care Patients for Depression?" *American Journal of Hospice and Palliative Care* 19 (2002): 112–114.

Medical Treatment

Homsi, J., D. A. Nelson, N. Sarhill, L. Rybicki, S. B. LeGrand, M. P. Davis, and D. Walsh. "A Phase II Study of Methylphenidate for Depression in Advanced Cancer." *American Journal of Hospice and Palliative Care* 16 (2001): 403–407.

Pereira, J. and E. Bruera. "Depression with Psychomotor Retardation: Diagnostic Challenges and the Use of Psychostimulants." *Journal of Palliative Medicine* 4 (2001): 15–21.

Schwartz, L., M. Lander, and H. M. Chochinov. "Current Management of Depression in Cancer Patients." *Oncology* 16 (2002): 1102–1115.

3.4   Grief and Bereavement

Key Points

1. Grief is a universal response to any kind of loss.

    The grief response is emotional, cognitive, and behavioral. Examples of losses occasioning grief include loss of job, loss of friendship, loss of child departing for college, and loss of physical ability.

2. The experience of grief and loss is particularly complex and intense at Life's End.

    Everyone involved experiences grief: the dying person, the family and significant others, and caregivers and medical providers—including the physician.

3. Some persons may require intervention for complicated or pathological grief.

    Complicated grief is more intense, prolonged, and disabling and may endanger the bereaved person by becoming self-destructive. Manifestations include self-neglect, substance abuse or other harmful coping behaviors, depression, and suicidality. The Palliative Response to grief uses a multidisciplinary approach including pastoral care, counseling, and medical assessment to monitor the bereavement progress and to intervene in complicated grief.

4. We now know that the stages of loss described by Kubler-Ross are neither predictable nor neatly progressive.

    Manifestation of grief may oscillate back and forth between stages, and elements of different stages may occur simultaneously. "Getting stuck" in one stage of grief is a sign of complicated bereavement.

5. Normal grief includes an initial sense of disintegration—a period of feeling less whole and complete—followed by reintegration that incorporates the loss into one's sense of self.

6. Discussing honestly what is happening and what is likely to happen avoids mixed messages and allows the patient and family time for preparation.

    Patients need time to review their lives. Loved ones need to plan for a future without the patient. Honesty allows everyone to expect, understand, and prepare for losses and to attend to needs in all domains of suffering.

Grief and Bereavement

The Palliative Response

Grief Is Universal

- Grief is a response to loss
  Emotional response
  Cognitive response
  Behavioral response

- Grief is experienced with many kinds of losses
  Loss of job
  Loss of friendship following disagreement
  Loss of child departing for college
  Loss of physical ability

Grief and Loss at Life's End

- Particularly complex and intense
- Experienced by everyone involved
  Dying person
  Family
  Significant others
  Caregivers and medical providers, including physicians

Anticipatory Grief

- Who?
  Dying patient
  Loved ones

- When?
  Prior to death

- Why?
  In anticipation of the impending loss

Bereavement

- What?
  Grief
  Mourning

- Who?
  Family, friends, personal caregivers
  Medical professionals

- When?
  After the death of the patient/loved one

Complicated or Pathological Grief

Indications and manifestations
- More intense and prolonged
- Disabling (depression, self-neglect)
- Endangering (substance abuse, other harmful coping behaviors, suicidal)

Intervention
- Monitor progress of grief process
- Multidisciplinary approach usually indicated *(medical assessment, counseling, pastoral care)*

Dimensions of Grief

Presentation
- Sadness over loss
- Distinguished from depression (which is marked by lack of self-worth)
- Often comes in waves
- Triggers may or may not be predictable

Course
- Often very intense at first
- Intensity/frequency usually diminish over time

Stages of Grief

Interpretation of stages of grief
(described by Kubler-Ross)
- Stages are not predictable
- Manifestation may oscillate between stages
- Progression varies from person to person
- Elements of stages may occur simultaneously

Complicated grief
- Failure to progress through grief
- "Getting stuck" in one stage of grief

Effect of Grief on Sense of Self

Initial sense of disintegration
- Loss of any sort can affect sense of self
- Period of feeling less whole and complete
- Initial sense of disintegration

Process of reintegration
- Fostered by normal grief work
- Fashion a newly integrated self
- Experienced loss finds its place in one's sense of self

The Physician's Role
Honesty at Life's End

Truth-telling in diagnosis and prognosis
- Avoids mixed messages by discussing without ambiguity what is happening and likely to happen
- Allows patients to review their lives
- Assists loved ones to plan for a future that necessarily will be very different
- Allows everyone to expect, understand, prepare for loss
- Helps identify and attend to needs/suffering

Honesty Fosters Communication

Five things everyone needs to say at Life's End:

Forgive me
I forgive you
Thank you
I love you
Good bye

The Physician's Role
Open Communication

Fostering communication
- Open the door to discussion
- Then listen!

Conversation starters
- "Things have been changing. How are you and your family coping with the changes?"
- "Are you feeling afraid or overwhelmed?"

The Physician's Role
Assess/Treat

- What?
  Symptoms
- Why?
  Foster comfort for patient
  Free energy, and often more time, for patient and family to work through their grief and prepare for the loss of death
- How?
  Aggressively!

The Physician's Role
Familiarity with Resources

- Pastoral care
- Community support groups
- Communities of faith
- Counseling
- Grief and survivor's groups
- Social Work services
- Community mental-health providers

The Physician's Role
At Time of Death

- Respond empathically
  "I am sorry for your loss"
  Offer to call someone
- Be available
  Answer questions
  Give family and friends time to process
  Welcome contact with the family for future questions and needs
- Check back in

The Physician's Role
After the Death

- Offer emotional support
  Consider sending cards
  Offer to maintain dialogue with the family
- Offer practical support
  Write necessary letters
  Sign necessary forms
  Reassure family you will be helpful
- Offer availability
  Often nagging questions come up later

Bereavement
Follow-up Programs

- Who?
  Medicare hospice programs
  Palliative-care programs
- Why?
  Help facilitate grief work
  Monitor for complicated grief
- How long?
  Up to one year

Grief and Bereavement
The Palliative Response

Honesty at Life's End allows patient, family, friends, and medical caregivers to expect, understand, and prepare for the loss of death.

Grief and Bereavement

Selected Readings

Dying as a Process

Wade, D. T. "The Disintegration of Death." *The Lancet* 360 (2002): 425–426.

Family Experience

Billings, J. A. and E. Kolton. "Family Satisfaction and Bereavement Care Following Death in the Hospital." *Journal of Palliative Medicine* 2 (1999): 33–49.

Morita, T., S. Chihara, and T. Kashiwagi. "Quality Audit Committee of the Japanese Association of Hospice and Palliative Care Units: A Scale to Measure Satisfaction of Bereaved Family Receiving Inpatient Palliative Care." *Palliative Medicine* 16 (2002): 141–150.

Silverman, P. R. "Living with Grief, Rebuilding a World." *Journal of Palliative Medicine* 5 (2002): 449–454.

Teno, J. M., V. A. Casey, L. C. Welch, and S. Edgman-Levitan. "Patient-Focused, Family-Centered End-of-Life Medical Care: Views of the Guidelines and Bereaved Family Members." *Journal of Pain and Symptom Management* 22 (2001): 738–751.

Medical Provider Experience

Rosenblum, J. L. "Why I Still Cry. Share a Young Internist's Reflections on the Death of a Patient at the End of a Long Day." *Medical Economics Magazine* 79 (2002): 65–66.

Spiritual Suffering: The Palliative Response

4.1 Religious and Spiritual Issues: Assessing and Addressing

Key Points

1. Spiritual and religious concerns may develop or intensify at Life's End. Many patients welcome an opportunity to talk about spiritual issues in relation to their health and current life experience. Patients and families often avoid these issues for fear of upsetting each other; many physicians feel unskilled, unprepared, and uncomfortable talking to patients about their spiritual and existential concerns.

2. Use a format, such as "FICA," to elicit concerns and identify sources of support. Normalize the topic.
   Faith—Do you consider yourself a spiritual person?
   Importance—Is faith important to you?
   Community—Are you part of a spiritual or faith community?
   Address—How can I address and respect these issues in your care?

3. Share the patient's wondering and questioning and what it is like to be human and to face Life's End. Do not attempt to answer the unanswerable.

4. Elicit further concerns with open-ended questions.
   Do you have any thoughts about why this is happening to you (your family)?
   Help me understand what you mean.
   Many people with serious illnesses like yours ask such questions.
   That sounds kind of scary or troubling to me too.
   How does this make you feel?

5. Discussion guidelines
   • Empathize and share in the uncertainty;
   • Be guided by the patient's own search;
   • Answer personal questions simply; keep the focus on the patient;
   • Allow time and permission for expression of a range of emotions;
   • Clarify sources of hope, meaning, and support; identify Goals of Care that can help maintain hope; honor preferences at Life's End;
   • Foster religious participation and spiritual practice.

   Pitfalls include trying to "fix" patient's problem, imposing or debating personal religious beliefs, providing inappropriate reassurance, and failing to attend to physician's own faith in light of continued losses.

Religious and Spiritual Issues

The Palliative Response

Religion and Spirituality at Life's End

- Spiritual and religious concerns may develop or intensify at Life's End
- Many patients are thinking about these issues in relationship to their health
- Many patients welcome an opportunity to talk about religious and spiritual issues as they relate to their current life experience

Barriers to Addressing Religious and Spiritual Issues

- Many persons have not expressed their existential concerns at Life's End for fear of upsetting families and friends
- Many physicians feel unskilled, unprepared, and uncomfortable talking to patients about religious and spiritual concerns

Getting Started

- Ask open-ended questions
- Use a format
- Listen and respond empathically
- Be familiar with resources
  Pastoral care
  Social Work and counseling
  Communities of faith

The FICA Format*

- **F**aith
- **I**mportance
- **C**ommunity
- **A**ddress

Christina M. Puchalski, M.D., M.S., The George Washington Institute for Spirituality and Health

Faith

"Do you consider yourself a spiritual person?"

"Is faith important to you?"

- Most patients can answer this kind of question
- Include question in social history
- Normalize discussion of faith as part of routine and not a topic indicating that patient is "imminently dying"

Importance

"Is your faith important in your life at this time?"

"Have you been able to take comfort from your faith?"

- May reveal sources of strength and support
- May guide physician in assisting patient to maintain sources of support

Community

"Are you part of a spiritual or faith community?"

- May reveal a source of support
- May reveal that individual has become isolated from faith community

Frequent occurrence when chronic illness prevents participation in faith community

Physician may be able to foster re-connection

Address

"How can I address and respect these issues in your care?"

- Patient may have important beliefs, practices, and rituals that are not part of your tradition
- Understanding patient's tradition early on allows the physician to be sensitive to needs

Patient's Response

Many patients:

- Speak openly
- Are grateful to physician for asking about this important part of life
- Express no specific concerns or needs

When Patient Voices Concern

Respond with:

- Open-ended questions
- Comments to normalize the concern

"Help me understand what you mean."

"Many people with serious illnesses ask such questions."

"That sounds scary to me too."

"Do you have any thoughts about why this is happening to you (your family)?"

"How does this make you feel?"

Discussion Guideline
Share versus Fix

Do:

- Share patient's wondering and questioning
- Share in what it is like to be human and to face what is at Life's End

Do not:

- Do not try to resolve (fix) the patient's problem
- Do not try to answer unanswerable questions

Discussion Guideline
Follow versus Lead

Do:
- Stay within physician's role and expertise
- Be guided by patient's own search

Do not:
- Proselytize
- Try to convert a vulnerable individual
- Impose personal religious or spiritual beliefs

Discussion Guideline
Support versus Reassure

Do:
- Allow time and permission for people to express emotions
- Develop comfort with tears and range of feelings

Do not:
- Do not offer premature or inappropriate reassurance
- Do not be a phony

Discussion Guideline
Questions about Physician's Beliefs

- Answer simply
  "I would like to keep the focus on you rather than me"
  "I am a person of faith"
- Avoid a religious debate
- Most patients are grateful that physician is interested in this important part of who they are

Steps of Palliative Response
Assess

For patients with life-threatening and life-limiting illness

- Clarify sources of hope and meaning
- Identify Goals of Care
  Maintain hope
  Honor preferences at Life's End

Steps of Palliative Response
Support

- Mobilize resources
  Healthcare team
  Patient's community and community at large
- Patient's spiritual/religious practice
  Solace
  Meaning
  Hope
  Connection

Steps of Palliative Response
Self-Care for the Physician

- Develop healthy personal responses to experiencing the repeated loss of death
- Self-monitor and seek assistance as needed for:
  Depression
  Substance abuse
  Burn-out

Religious and Spiritual Issues: Assessing and Addressing

Selected Readings

Religion and Spirituality at Life's End

Daaleman, T. P. and L. van de Creek. "Placing Religion and Spirituality in End-of-life Care." *Journal of the American Medical Association* 284 (2000): 2514–2517.

Rousseau, P. "Spirituality and the Dying Patient." *Journal of Clinical Oncology* 18 (2000): 2000–2002.

Professional Considerations for Physicians

Post, S. G., C. M. Puchalski, and D. B. Larson. "Physicians and Patient Spirituality: Professional Boundaries, Competency, and Ethics." *Annals of Internal Medicine* 132 (2000): 578–583.

Listening and Caring/FICA

Puchalski, C. M. "Spirituality and End-of-life Care: A Time for Listening and Caring." *Journal of Palliative Medicine* 5 (2002): 289–294.

Redefining Hope

Parker-Oliver, D. "Redefining Hope for the Terminally Ill." *American Journal of Hospice and Palliative Care* 19 (2002): 115–120.

4.2 Spiritual Distress: Fostering Transcendence at Life's End

Key Points

1. Spiritual questions are common at Life's End and a major source of distress for some persons.

   The spiritual dimension is broader than formal religious beliefs and includes existential questions concerning "why things happen." Most patients think about spiritual issues and are open to discussing them with medical providers.

2. Individuals at Life's End often struggle to maintain connections and to achieve a sense of transcendence over death.

   Transcendence is an achieved state of meaning and hope, providing connections with family and others across life-changing events and ultimately even death itself.

3. Life's End threatens the sources of meaning by which persons have defined themselves.

   Examples of sources of meaning are family, children, religious faith, career, patriotism and country, friends and community, material possessions, pets, hobbies, causes, civic clubs, party affiliations, the arts, and nature.

4. Patients often struggle to maintain meaningful roles even when they can no longer perform them effectively.

   The palliative response to this struggle is to assist the person to reframe and explore sources of meaning and to strengthen, maintain, and develop connections.

5. The palliative response to spiritual distress includes acknowledging, normalizing, and discussing the distress while responding effectively to all forms of suffering.

   Truth-telling helps individuals decide how to plan and prioritize family and other responsibilities. Attempting to shield people from "harsh" reality may lead them to put off work and activities important to them. Refer to pastoral care and/or the faith community as appropriate for each individual.

6. Assist with spiritual distress by reframing the process of "helping" to a focus on supporting.

   Support with truth and honesty. Support to live life fully. Support to live with joy, expectation, and hope. It is not within our power to do this for others; rather, we must support people as they find their way.

Spiritual Distress

The Palliative Response

Spiritual Questioning at Life's End

- Common

  Most patients have been thinking about spiritual issues and are open to discussion with physician

- Can be a major source of distress

- Existential

  Why things happen

  Not answered by science and medicine, which address how things happen

  Extends beyond formal religious beliefs

Fostering Transcendence

- Transcendence is a state of meaning and hope providing connection with family and others:

  across life-changing events

  ultimately across even death itself

- Individuals at Life's End often struggle:

  to maintain connections

  to achieve a sense of transcendence

Examples of Transcendence

- If a member of your family has died, do you still consider this person a part of your family?

- If so, you have achieved some degree of transcendence over death, since you are maintaining a connection with the person who has died

Life as Defined by Meaning

Examples of things that give life meaning:

Family

Children

Religious faith

Career

Patriotism and country

Friends and community

Life as Defined by Meaning

The list continues:

Material possessions

Pets

Hobbies

Causes, civic clubs, party affiliations

The arts—music, literature, visual arts

Nature

Life's End Often Threatens Our Sources of Meaning

"Everyone wants to go to heaven, but no one wants to die to get there."

—H.L. Mencken

Changing Relationship to Sources of Meaning

The patient's struggle

- To find meaning when he can no longer maintain roles that gave life meaning
- May attempt to maintain meaningful roles beyond ability to perform them

The palliative response

- Reframe and explore sources of meaning
- Strengthen, maintain, develop connections

Suffering with Loss of Sources of Meaning

"The state of severe distress associated with events that threaten the intactness of a person."

—E. Cassell, 1991

Spiritual/Existential Distress The Palliative Response

Ask and listen

- Accept and normalize
- Acknowledge spiritual distress
- Confirm distress as part of suffering at Life's End

Explore

- Be willing and available to discuss spiritual issues

- Help patient incorporate this aspect of personhood into current life and illness

Rx for Spiritual Distress
Tell the Truth

- Offer honest assessment of probable prognosis and course of illness
- Helps patient/family plan and prioritize
- Attempting to shield people from "harsh" reality may result in their inability to accomplish important work of Life's End

Rx for Spiritual Distress
Help Patient Prioritize

- Which is more important?

  Staying in town to take chemo–therapy for stage IV lung cancer?

  or

  Visiting a daughter in another state who has just delivered a new grandchild?

- *Tuesdays with Morrie* shows how an individual may actively "live" at Life's End

Rx for Spiritual Distress
Respond to All Suffering

- Excellent symptom control

  Frees time and energy to work out issues
- Community resources

  Assistance to maintain efficacy at Life's End (e.g., hospice)
- Pastoral counseling

  Refer to pastoral care and/or faith community as appropriate for each individual

Rx for Spiritual Distress
Reframe "Helping"

Help as <u>support</u>

- <u>Support</u> with truth and honesty
- <u>Support</u> to live life fully
- <u>Support</u> to live with joy, expectation, hope

Rx for Spiritual Distress
Reframe "Helping"

Help as <u>support</u> versus <u>fix:</u>

- Not within our power resolve spiritual issues for others
- Must support people to find their way

Rx for Spiritual Distress
Help Patient Leave Legacies

- Write letters and make videos (especially for children too young to remember)
- Tell and write stories
- Make scrapbooks
- Distribute personal belongings, mementos, or heirlooms

Rx for Spiritual Distress
Help Patient Make Memories

- Celebrate birthdays and holidays "out of season"
- Family reunions and get-togethers
- Physician can assist with time off from work for family

Spiritual Distress

Selected Readings

Spirituality and Health

Puchalski, C. M. "Touching the Spirit: The Essence of Healing." *Spiritual Life* 1999 (Fall): 154–159.

Overview of Religion and Spirituality at Life's End

Koenig, H. G. "The Role of Religion and Spirituality at the End of Life." *The Gerontologist* 42 (2002): 20–23.

Transcendence at Life's End

Block, S. D. "Psychological Considerations, Growth, and Transcendence at the End of Life." *Journal of the American Medical Association* 285 (2001): 2898–2905.

Byock, I. "The Meaning and Value of Death." *Journal of Palliative Medicine* 4 (2002): 279–288.

Discussing Religious and Spiritual Issues at Life's End

Lo, B., D. Ruston, L. W. Kates, et. al. "Discussing Religious and Spiritual Issues at the End of Life: A Practical Guide for Physicians." *Journal of the American Medical Association* 287 (2002): 749–754.

Procedures

at Life's End

5.1 Sharing Bad News

Key Points

1. Patients and families want and need to know the truth of their situation.

    Patients and families need to plan location and contingencies of physical care; understand Goals of Care in the social, emotional, and spiritual areas of suffering; and strengthen their therapeutic relationship with the physician.

2. Carefully plan sharing bad news. Set the stage for an effective conversation.

    Sharing bad news is a part of the physician's role that should not be delegated. Confirm medical facts and plan to present only one or two main points in simple language. Choose an appropriate and private environment; determine who should be present; and allot a minimum of 30 minutes for the conversation.

3. Begin a conversation by asking the patient or family how they understand what is going on. Use silence to encourage dialogue.

    Ask the patient and family what others have told them and how they understand the situation. Sit quietly for 15–30 seconds to allow response.

4. Patients usually want to know the truth. Some families wish to "protect" the patient from the truth.

    Patient may prefer to designate a spokesperson. Physician goals are to honor patient autonomy, meet the legal obligation for patient consent, and promote family alliance and support for the patient. Interventions include querying the family about fears and offering to include them in the conversation with the patient.

5. Do not minimize the severity of the bad news.

    If "this is an illness that man cannot cure," say so. Remain humble. Assist the patient and family to change the focus from cure to palliation and support, while leaving open the possibility of the miraculous.

6. Respond to the emotional reaction of patient, family, and staff.

    Allow time for response. Offer follow-up meeting within 24 hours to repeat news and share it with absent family members. Offer to contact absent members and get permission to share the news if appropriate.

7. Briefly review the plan of care.

    Outline plan for medical and ancillary care. Suggest flexible timeline for upcoming decisions.

Sharing Bad News

The Palliative Response

Sharing Bad News
First Step in Planning Care

Helps develop therapeutic relationship

- Discuss agenda of patient/family first
- Let the physician priorities flow naturally from the patient/family (e.g., discussion of resuscitation and other advance directives)

Discussion Agenda

Physical care
- Setting and level of residential care

Social care
- Family issues (e.g., dependence)
- Financial issues (e.g., disability)

Emotional care
- Sources of support

Spiritual care
- Sources of meaning

Physician Preparation

- Confirm medical facts
- Plan presentation
  Make only one or two main points
  Use simple, lay language

"Your cancer has spread to the liver"
  versus
"You have hepatic metastatic disease from non-small cell lung cancer"

Physician's Role

DO NOT DELEGATE sharing bad news!

- Sharing bad news is physician's role
- Patients often accept bad news only from M.D.
- The physician is best prepared to interpret news and to offer advice

---

Setting the Stage

- Choose appropriate, private environment
  Neither hallway nor curtain provide privacy!
  Have tissue available
- Allot enough time (20–30 minutes minimum with documentation)
- Determine who should be present

Gathering

- Introduce yourself to everyone in the room
- Shake hands with patient first
- Turn beeper to vibrate to avoid interruptions and demonstrate full attention

Seating

- Always sit
  Eye level with patient
  Distance of 50–75cm
  Ask permission before sitting on edge of bed
- Arrange seating for everyone present if possible
  Helps put patient at ease
  Helps prevent patient from hurrying for others' comfort

Starting the Conversation

- Ask
  How do patient/family understand what is happening? What have others told them?
- Wait 15–30 seconds to give opportunity for response
  Elicit conversation versus physician monologue
- Listen
  Response may vary from "I think I am dying" to "I don't understand what is happening"
  Allow patient to talk further if he wishes.

How Much Does Patient Want to Know?

- Ask patient if he wants to know prognosis
  Patients usually want to know the truth
  May decline discussion and designate another person to be their spokesperson
- Factors determining desire to know
  Age
  Cultural background
  Capacity—emotional, educational, intellectual

When Family Wants to "Protect" Patient

- Physician goals for openness
  Honor patient's autonomy
  Meet legal obligation for consent
  Promote family alliance and support for the patient
- Physician interventions
  Ask what family is afraid will happen
  Offer to have family present when you speak to the patient so they can hear patient's wishes about knowing status/prognosis

Sharing the Bad News

- Give a warning to allow people to prepare
  "I wanted to talk to you about those X-rays we ordered yesterday…"
- Briefly state only key points
  Usually only one or two key points
  Use simple language

STOP:

Ask questions to assess understanding.

Do Not Minimize Severity of News

- Recommended statement for terminal illness:
  "This is an illness that man cannot cure"
- Humble statement
- Leaves open the possibility of the miraculous
- Helps change the focus from "cure" to palliation and support

Respond to Emotions of Patient, Family, Staff

- Be prepared for range of emotions
  Fear
  Anger
  Relief
  Denial (very rare)
  Emotional outburst
- Key components of response
  Allow time for response—Answer questions
  Communicate nonverbally as well as verbally—usually acceptable is to touch patient's <u>arm.</u>

Offer Follow-up Meeting

- When?
  Usually within 24 hours
- Who?
  Current and additional family members
- Why?
  To repeat portions of the news
- How?
  Offer to contact absent family members
  Get permission to share news if necessary

Suggest a Brief Plan

- Medical plan
  (e.g., control dyspnea, home assistance to help deal with weakness)
- Ancillary support
  (e.g., social work visits, pastoral care visits)
- Introduce advance care planning
  "Sometimes when people die, doctors try to bring them back to life...have you considered whether you would want this or not?"

Discuss Timeline

- Next meeting
  Review agenda
- Upcoming decisions
  Suggest flexible timeline

Ending the Meeting

- Ask
  "Do you have any questions?"
- Wait
- Answer
- Stand
  An effective way to end the conversation

Sharing Bad News

Selected Readings

<u>Overview of Physician Discussions at Life's End</u>

Lo, B., T. E. Quill, and J. Tulsky. "Discussing Palliative Care with Patients." *Annals of Internal Medicine* 130 (1999): 744–749.

Buckman, R. "Communication in Palliative Care: A Practical Guide" In *Oxford Textbook of Palliative Medicine,* edited by D. Doyle, G. W. Hanks, and N. MacDonald. Oxford Univeristy Press, 141–156.

Quill, T. E. "Initiating End-of-life Discussions with Seriously Ill Patients: Addressing the "Elephant in the Room." *Journal of the American Medical Association* 284 (2000): 2502–2507.

<u>Specific Aspects of Physician Discussions at Life's End</u>

Back, A. L., R. M. Arnold, and T. E. Quill. "Hope for the Best and Prepare for the Worst." *Annals of Internal Medicine* 138 (2003): 439–443.

Quill, T. E., R. M. Arnold, and E. Platt. "I Wish Things Were Different." *Annals of Internal Medicine* 135 (2001): 551–555.

Stolick, M. "Overcoming the Tendency to Lie to Dying Patients." *American Journal of Hospice and Palliative Care* 19 (2002): 29–34.

<u>Patient Preferences for Communication with Physicians</u>

Hofmann, J. C., N. S. Wenger, R. B. Davis, J. Teno, et al. "Patient Preferences for Communication with Physicians about End-of-life Decisions." *Annals of Internal Medicine* 127 (1997): 1–12.

5.2 Goals of Care

Key Points

1. Helping patients identify, express, and achieve their Goals of Care is a key role for the physician. Aids include reviewing sources of personal meaning, convening family conferences, and considering hospice and palliative care.

2. Open discussion is the key to helping choose the best pathway for the patient.
   - Review the current clinical condition with the patient as an introduction to identifying, prioritizing, and setting Goals of Care.
   - Discuss Goals of Care (medical, social, emotional, and spiritual) in the context of the prognosis. If it is true, say something like, "This is an illness that man cannot cure" to steer the conversation to Goals of Care other than cure.
   - The physician may propose as Goals of Care better symptom control, improvement of function, care at home, time with family and friends, and avoidance of unwanted and potentially burdensome interventions.
   - Respond to unrealistic or illegal goals by making the conflict explicit, setting limits without implying abandonment, and offering to assist in other ways.

3. Truth-telling is crucial at Life's End. Honesty allows patients and families to understand the seriousness of the situation so that they can address important issues they might otherwise neglect. In discussing prognosis:
   - Acknowledge uncertainty and pace the conversation;
   - Use a range of time to predict life expectancy;
   - Choose language carefully to avoid unintended meanings.
   Never say:
   "to withdraw care"
   "There is nothing left to do."
   "I think it is time to stop aggressive care."
   "I am asking you to agree to stop care."
   "Do you still want us to do everything?"
   Instead, say:
   "We will always care for you (your loved one)."
   "Sometimes the burden of therapy outweighs the benefit."

4. Focusing on the possible in the face of the impossible can help patients and providers find meaning, hope, and satisfaction in the midst of broken situations.

Goals of Care

The Palliative Response

Goals of Care
Parameters

Who?

- Helping patients identify, express, and achieve their Goals of Care is a key role for the physician

Why?

- Defining Goals of Care can help patient, family, and medical providers choose wisely among the options for medical care

When?

- Goals of Care change over time and must be reassessed

Communication about Goals

Language

- Physician must use language carefully to communicate and work together effectively with patients

Patient-centered goal setting

- Goals are often multiple and even contradictory
- Physician can help patient identify, prioritize, and achieve Goals of Care

Exploring Patient's Sense of Meaning

- Who am I?
- What are my roles?
- What do I like and dislike?
- What do I hope for?
- What gives me joy or meaning?
- What do I fear?

Open Discussion Is Vital

Importance of open discussion that may be outside of the routine physician-patient discussion

- Understand what is important to the patient
- Build trust
- Identify sources of support
- Key to helping choose the best pathway for the patient

Review Current
Clinical Condition

- Ask patient to describe understanding of illness and treatment plan
  Always a good idea
  Even though physician may have already stated diagnosis and prognosis
- Restate the key healthcare issues, especially if:
  Time has elapsed since last discussion
  New people are part of the discussion

Discussing Goals in Context of Prognosis

State the truth

- If it is true, it is good to say something like…

  "This is an illness man cannot cure"

- Advantage of this statement

  Humble

  Leaves open the possibility of the miraculous

  Clear language

  Helps steer the conversation to Goals of Care other than cure

Possible Goals of Care
Medical

- Cure of disease
- Good Quality of Life
- Maximum quantity of life
- Improvement of function
- Better symptom control
- Sense of personal control

Possible Goals of Care
Social-Emotional-Spiritual

- Location of care other than hospital or nursing home
- Support for family and loved ones
- Making memories with friends and family
- Creating a legacy
- "Taking care of business"
- "Getting things in order"
- Reconciliation—making peace

Palliative Care
Ideal for Complex Goals

- Interdisciplinary
- Symptom-focused
- Access to maximum support not always available in settings of treatment

  Hospital

  Home

  Nursing home

Truth-Telling

- Prognostication is hard

  Physicians typically overestimate survival

- Honesty is important at Life's End

  Allows patients and families to understand seriousness of situation

  Fosters addressing, rather than neglecting, important issues

- Offer both honesty and hope

  Skillful clinician can be honest while helping find hope for realistic Goals of Care

Discussing Prognosis

- Acknowledge uncertainty

  Explain that unexpected events can change prognosis

  Offer to be honest and inform patients of changes in status as they wish

- Pace the conversation

  Allow people time to respond

  Be led by desire for information and ability to process it

Discussing Life Expectancy

Best to use a range of time when making a prognosis:

Hours to days
Days to weeks
Weeks to months
Months to years

The Palliative Response

Avoiding Unintended Meanings
Choice of Language

- We will always care for you (your loved one)
- Sometimes the burden of a therapy outweighs the benefit
- Never say…
  Withdraw care
  There is nothing left to do
  I think it is time to stop aggressive care
  I am asking you to agree to stop care
  Do you still want us to do everything?

Suggesting Goals of Care

- Better control of symptoms
- Care at home when appropriate
- Time with family and friends
- Avoidance of unwanted and potentially burdensome treatments/interventions
- Improvement in function

Aids to Suggesting Goals of Care

- Review sources of personal meaning
  Identify goals
  Prioritize goals
  Choose goals
- Convene a family conference
  Can help resolve differences in Goals of Care between patient, family, and providers
- Consider hospice/palliative care
  May provide resources to achieve goals

When Goals Are Unrealistic or Illegal

- Make the conflict explicit
  I understand that you want to live alone…
  But I cannot send you to an unsafe place
- Set limits without implying abandonment
  I understand that you were hoping to have surgery to remove the tumor…
  But the surgeons are saying it is not physically possible
  Are there other ways we can help you with this problem?

Goals of Care
Reframe and Foster Hope

Focusing on the possible in the face of the impossible can help patients and providers find meaning, hope, and satisfaction in the midst of broken situations.

Goals of Care

Selected Readings

Overview of Palliative Goals

Bruera, E. and C. M. Neumann. "Management of Specific Symptom Complexes in Patients Receiving Palliative Care." *Canadian Medical Association Journal* 158 (1998): 1717–1726.

O'Brien, T., J. Welsh, and F. G. Dunn. "ABC of Palliative Care: Non-malignant Conditions." *British Medical Journal* 316 (1998): 286–289.

Establishing Goals of Care

Phillips, R. S., M. B. Hamel, J. M. Teno, J. Soukup, J. Lynn, R. Califf, H. Vidaillet, R. B. Davis, P. Bellamy, and L. Goldman. "Patient Race and Decisions to Withhold or Withdraw Life-sustaining Treatments for Seriously Ill Hospitalized Adults." SUPPORT Investigators. Study to Understand Prognoses and Preferences for Outcomes and Risks of Treatments. *American Journal of Medicine* 108: 9–14.

Stevens, L., D. Cook, G. Guyatt, L. Griffith, S. Walter, and J. McMullin. "Education, Ethics, and End-of-life Decisions in the Intensive Care Unit." *Critical Care Medicine* 30 (2002): 290–296.

Teno, J. M., D. Murphy, J. Lynn, A. Tosteson, N. Desbiens, A. F. Connors Jr., M. B. Hamel, A. Wu, R. Philllips, N. Wenger et al. "Prognosis-based Futility Guidelines: Does Anyone Win?" SUPPORT Investigators. Study to Understand Prognoses and Preferences for Outcomes and Risks of Treatment." *Journal of the American Geriatrics Society* 42: 1202–1207.

Vigano, A., M. Dorgan, E. Bruera, and M. E. Suarez-Almazor. "The Relative Accuracy of the Clinical Estimation of the Duration of Life for Patients with End-of-life Cancer." *Cancer* 86 (199):170–176.

Goals Regarding Site of Death

Middlewood, S., G. Gardner, and A. Gardner. "Dying in Hospital: Medical Failure or Natural Outcome?" *Journal of Pain and Symptom Management* 22 (6): 1035–1041.

Physician-Family Communication

Limerick, M. "Communicating with Surrogate Decision-makers in End-of-life Situations: Substitutive Descriptive Language for the Healthcare Provider." *American Journal of Hospice and Palliative Care* 19 (2002): 376–380.

5.3 Advance Care Planning

Key Points

1. The advance directive (AD) is a valuable clinical and personal tool.
   The AD helps the physician build trust, assist the patient to plan future care, designate a proxy decision-maker, and explore values and fears relating to health care. It allows patients to reduce uncertainty, avoid family conflicts, and achieve peace of mind.

2. Discussion of advance directives should be a routine part of care.
   Physicians should discuss AD as routinely as any other health promotion or prevention issue. Barriers to successful use include physician discomfort and time pressure, poor timing of discussion, and the cumbersome legal language of some documents.

3. Physicians should carefully plan discussion about advance directives.
   An AD discussion should include:
   - Designation of surrogate
   - Documentation of healthcare preferences
   - Review of the AD document
   - Encouragement to discuss AD with family
   - Scheduling future time to review completed document and address questions
   - A plan for distribution of document to surrogate, family members, physicians, and faith community representative

4. Physicians should periodically review advance directive with patient.
   Indications for future review and modification of AD include a major change in patient's health status and/or a change in the health status or availability of the designated surrogate.

5. Advance directives are not equivalent to DNAR orders.
   AD may specify various degrees of aggressiveness of treatment.

Advance Care Planning

The Palliative Response

Advance Directives
Frequency of Use

- The Federal Patient Self Determination Act mandates that all hospital admissions include information on Advance Directives (AD)
- Still, relatively few persons have completed an AD
- Studies show that the physician is frequently unaware of an AD, if it exists

Advance Directive as a Clinical Tool

- Plan and document preferences for future medical care
- Designate proxy decision-maker
- Explore values, fears, and other concerns
- Foster trust with provider

Advance Directive as a Personal Tool

- Build trust
- Define and document goals
- Reduce uncertainty
- Avoid family conflicts
- Permit peace of mind

Advance Care Planning
Barriers to Success

- Physician reluctance
  Personal discomfort
  Time pressure
- Poor timing
  Crisis situation vs. during clinic visit or at hospital discharge
- Cumbersome language

Advance Care Planning
Component of Basic Care

- Include AD as part of clinical routine
  "I encourage all of my patients to complete an Advance Directive"
- Patient is less likely to be alarmed or to fear that provider anticipates imminent death if Advance Planning is routine

Advance Care Planning
Getting Started

- Introduce topic in least stressful setting

  Clinic visit

  Hospital discharge planning
- Use natural language and approach

  "You were pretty sick when you came to the hospital. If you got so sick that you couldn't speak for yourself...

  • Who would you want to speak for you?

  • What would you want them to know?"

Advance Care Planning
Discuss Naturally and Calmly

- Discuss Advance Planning as you would any health promotion or prevention issue

  Similar to tobacco cessation intervention
- Be observant about patient's comfort level
- Extend conversation into future visits

  Follow up, give homework, encourage, praise success

The Planning Document
Introduce as Advance Directive rather than Living Will

- Patient less likely to be familiar with AD
- Allows physician to define instrument
- Distinguishes from Living Will

  "Have you heard about advance directives?

  Let me tell you a little bit about them"

Designation of Surrogate

- Patient's preferred decision-maker
- Good opening question
- Less threatening than healthcare decisions
- Documentation especially important if patient prefers a surrogate outside the usual legal progression (e.g., patient names domestic partner or friend rather than spouse or children)

Healthcare Preferences
Discussing and Documenting

"If something happened and you could not speak for yourself... your surrogate might have to make difficult decisions."

"It is helpful to discuss the kinds of treatment you might want or not want...and to write down some things to guide that person."

Review and Complete

- Review an advance directive document (e.g., *The Five Wishes*)
- Demonstrate briefly how to complete
- Encourage discussion of AD with family
- Plan to meet again to review the document and answer questions

Documentation

- Copy completed AD for patient's chart

  Write Advance Directive note to alert others

  If you do not document, it did not happen!

- Suggest that patient/family keep copies
- Remind patient/family to inform providers of AD at ER visits/ hospital admissions

Indication for Review
Change in Status of Patient

- Major change in patient's health
- Change in treatment preference
- "I wanted to go on the vent for my COPD if necessary, but since I have learned about the cancer, I feel different."

Indication for Review
Change in Status of Surrogate

- Death
- Relocation
- Cognitive impairment
- "My wife has had a stroke; I don't think she could be my surrogate anymore."

Advance Directives
Utilization

- Assure that <u>physicians</u> are aware of the existence of Advance Directive
- Read and discuss the AD with <u>surrogate</u>
- Consider an Ethics Committee consult if problems arise about interpreting AD
- Carry out the plan of the AD

AD versus DNAR

- An AD is <u>not</u> equivalent to a Do Not Attempt to Resuscitate (DNAR) order
- The AD may specify a variety of different degrees of aggressiveness of therapy

Encourage Non-Medical Planning

- Location of care
- Autopsy
- Funeral plans
- Guardianship for children or other dependents
- Plans for pets
- Financial arrangements
- Gifts
- Disposition of personal belongings

Advance Care Planning

Selected Readings

Physician Experience

Derse, A. R. "Decision-Making Capacity: Determination and Consequences." *Supportive Oncology Updates* 2 (1), 1999.

Tulsky, J. A., G. S. Fischer, M. R. Rose, and R. M. Arnold. "Opening the Black Box: How Do Physicians Communicate about Advance Directives?" *Annals of Internal Medicine* 129 (1998): 441–449.

Patient Experience

Kuczewski, M. "Cancer Patients Say the Darnedest Things: Commentary on "Paradoxes in Cancer Patients' Advance Care Planning." *Journal of Palliative Medicine* 3 (2000): 23–35.

Evolution of Palliative Medicine

Baumrucker, S. "AND versus DNR." *American Journal of Hospice and Palliative Care* 18 (2001): 370–371.

Ditillo, B. A. "Should There Be a Choice for Cardiopulmonary Resuscitation when Death Is Expected? Revisiting an Old Idea whose Time Is Yet to Come." *Journal of Palliative Medicine* 5 (2002): 107–116.

Tolle, S. W. and V. P. Tilden. "Changing End-of-life Planning: The Oregon Experience." *Journal of Palliative Medicine* 5 (2002): 311–317.

5.4 Family Conferences

Key Points

1. The family conference is often the key palliative care "procedure."
   A conference can be very therapeutic for the patient and family and helps the medical team identify sources of support for the patient. Time invested early reaps great benefits.

2. Careful preparation is the key to success.
   - Choose private space with ample seating.
   - Recruit appropriate members of the medical team to be present.
   - "Family" are those who claim to be family; include as many members as want to and can attend.
   - Include the patient if able and wishes to participate.
   - Otherwise, ask patient's permission to discuss care.
   - Schedule 30–60 min. minimum at a time convenient for family.

3. Solicit family understanding of illness. Offer to give your understanding of the problem. Focus on two to three key problems.
   - Use silence to allow family to respond.
   - Respond empathically.
   - Use simple language and avoid jargon.
   - If true, say "Your Aunt May has an illness man cannot cure."

4. Begin to define and establish with family the Goals of Care. Direct attention away from cure toward symptom management. Present a plan based on Goals of Care.
   - Discuss combination of disease modification and palliative treatment.
   - Explicitly state plan for symptom control and discuss avoidance of invasive medical procedures.
   - Explain how each member of interdisciplinary team will work with family to achieve the Goals of Care.

5. Discuss advance directive and other aggressive care options in light of whether they advance the Goals of Care.
   - Emphasize desire to honor the treatment preferences of patient and family.
   - Education about the effectiveness and process of resuscitation can be helpful.
   - Take as much responsibility on yourself as you can for making medical care decisions.
   - Avoid making families feel that they are responsible for "pulling the plug."
   - Demonstrate nonabandonment by clarifying that your support is not contingent on family decisions about "code status."
   - Review decisions. Allow time for questions and make sure people have contact numbers.

6. Document who was present, length of conference, and Goals of Care.

Family Conferences

The Palliative Response

Importance of Family Conference

Often the key palliative care "procedure"

- Can be very therapeutic for patient and family
- Helps medical team identify sources of support for the patient
- Time invested early reaps great benefits

Preparation

- Choose private space with seating
- Recruit appropriate members of the medical team to be present
- Remember that the idea of a family conference can be frightening

  Providers seldom call a conference for "good news"

Participants

- Family is who claims to be family

  "Aunt" who is not a blood relative may have raised patient or lived in the household

  As many members as want to and can attend

- Patient

  If able and wishes to participate

  Ask permission to discuss care

- Schedule at time convenient for family (30–60 minutes minimum)

Consideration of Spokesperson

- Some clinicians recommend that communication be through a family spokesperson
- Many minority cultures make family decisions by consensus of extended family vs. by single individual

Getting Started

- Identify relationships
- Ask family how they understand the illness
- Use silence to allow family to respond

  Usually natural spokesperson(s) will be apparent

- Respond empathically

  Offer to give your understanding of the problem

Focus on 2–3 Key Problems

- Use simple language and avoid jargon

  "Your Aunt May has an illness man cannot cure...."
- Identify current disease-modifying treatment and relative effectiveness
- Begin to to define Goals of Care

  Direct attention away from cure toward symptom management

Establish Goals of Care

- Combination of disease modification and palliative treatment

  Symptom control

  Avoidance of invasive medical procedures
- Time with family
- Care in the home

Present Plan of Care

- Present plan based on Goals of Care
- Explicitly state plan for symptom control
- Explain how each member of interdisciplinary team will work with family to achieve Goals of Care

  PT/OT

  Dietary

  Nurse case management

  Social work

  Pastoral care

Discussion

- Allow time for discussion
- Reassure that not all decisions need to be made at this time
- Discuss plan for follow-up and contact

Advance Care Planning
Introduction

Discuss

- Range of possible outcomes
- Problems that may arise and possible responses
- Desire to honor treatment preferences of patient and family
- Issues of resuscitation and other aggressive care options in light of whether they advance the Goals of Care

Discussing "Code Status"

Education about the effectiveness and process of resuscitation can be helpful

Sometimes when people are very ill, they die...

Sometimes the doctors and nurses try to bring people back to life with machines...

With the kind of illness Aunt May has, this is not a successful type of treatment...

Many patients and families discuss this kind of treatment with their doctors...

Discuss Alternatives

- Always emphasize what can and will be done to help patient
- Demonstrate non-abandonment
  Clarify that the your support is not contingent on family decisions about "code status"

Advance Care Planning

- Take as much responsibility on yourself as you can for making medical care decision
- Avoid making families feel that they are responsible for "pulling the plug"
- Offer ongoing support to families
- Offer to contact pastoral care or other resources

Documentation

- Document who was present
- Document length of conference
- List the Goals of Care
- Describe the plan of care

If no documentation, it didn't happen.

Documentation

- "With your permission, I am going to write a note and orders about our discussion and the decision we have made...."
- Review decisions
- Allow time for questions and make sure people have contact numbers

Implementation of Plan

- Monitor
- Make any conflicts explicit
  Suggest options and solutions
  Allow-patients and families to choose
- If Goal of Care is not achievable, state clearly

Family Conference
A Palliative Response

The family conference is often the key palliative care "procedure."

Handle with care.

Selected Readings

Family Perspective on Care at Life's End

Andrews, S. C. "Caregiver Burden and Symptom Distress in People with Cancer Receiving Hospice Care." *Oncology Nursing Forum* 28 (2001): 1469–1474.

Rao, J. and V. R. Koppaka. "On Being a Patient: Santi." *Annals of Internal Medicine* 137 (2002): 852–854.

Overview of Communication in End-of-Life Care

Faulkner, A. "ABC of Palliative Care: Communication with Patients, Families and Other Professionals." *British Medical Journal* 316 (1998): 130–132.

Conducting a Family Conference

Ambuel, B. "Conducting a Family Conference." In *Principles and Practice of Supportive Oncology* edited by A. M. Berger, R. K. Portenoy, and D. E. Weissman. New York: Lippincott Williams & Wilkins Healthcare, 3 (2000): 1–12.

Resolving Conflict and Making Decisions

Fins, J. J. and S. MZ. "Communication in Intensive Care Settings: The Challenge of Family Disputes." *Critical Care Medicine* 29 (2001): 1–10.

Glajchem, M. and C. Zuckerman. "Resolving Conflict and Making Decisions." *Journal of Palliative Medicine* 4 (2001): 221–225.

5.5 Subcutaneous Therapy

Key Points

1. Subcutaneous therapy offers an alternative to intravenous therapy.
   The SQ line is easier and less painful to place and has less risk of infection than the IV line. It is easy to use at home, gives the patient more freedom and control, and eliminates the need for painful and frequent IM injections.

2. SQ therapy offers an alternative to oral medications.
   SQ lines are useful when patients cannot take medications orally because of nausea/vomiting, delirium, seizures, changing level of consciousness, dysphagia, or esophageal obstruction.

3. SQ lines offer many clinical advantages in the palliative setting.
   The SQ line can be used for intermittent or continuous infusions to supply constant plasma levels, avoid first-pass metabolism, and present less danger of overhydration. All licensed nurses (both RN and LPN) can use SQ lines.

4. Disadvantages of SQ lines include inflammation at infusion site, logistical burdens, clinical limitations, and relative contraindications.
   Logistical burdens include necessity for needles, syringes, and possibly pumps, as well as nursing and pharmacy backup. Some medications and treatments cannot be given SQ. Relative contraindications include severe thrombocytopenia and edema.

5. Proper placement of an SQ line includes specific procedures for explaining, prepping, priming, inserting, securing, injecting, flushing, checking, and changing.
   Explain procedure to patient. See handout for complete description of the placement and care of SQ Line.

6. Appropriate medications for an SQ line include opioids, antiemetics, sedatives/anticonvulsants, corticosteroids, H2 blockers, antihistimine, hormones, and diuretics.
   Opioids used in SQ lines include morphine and hydomorphone. See handout for complete list of appropriate medications for SQ therapy.

7. Inappropriate medications for use in SQ lines include chlorpromazine (thorazine), prochlorperazine (compazine), and diazepam.

Subcutaneous Therapy

The Palliative Response

Alternative to Intravenous Therapy

- Easier to place
- Less painful to place
- Less risk of infection
- Easy to use at home
- Gives patient more freedom and control
- Eliminates need for painful and frequent IM injections

Alternative to Oral Medications

- Nausea and vomiting
- Last days of life
- Delirium
- Seizures
- Changing level of consciousness
- Dysphagia
- Esophageal obstruction

Clinical Advantages

- Can be used for intermittent or continuous infusions
- Provide constant plasma levels
- Avoids first-pass metabolism
- All licensed nurses (both RN and LPN) can use
- Less danger of overhydration

Clinical Advantages

- Avoids problems secondary to continuous IV fluids
  Edema
  Ascetes
  Pleural effusion
  Pulmonary congestion
- Hypodermoclysis
  May provide parentral hydration, when appropriate, with normal saline

Disadvantages

- Side effects
  May cause inflammation at infusion site
- Logistics
  Requires needles, syringes and possibly pumps
  Requires nursing and pharmacy backup

Disadvantages

- Clinical limitations
  Some medications/treatments cannot be given SQ
- Relative contraindications
  Severe thrombocytopenia
  Severe edema

Placing a SQ Line
Sites

- Bed-confined patients
  Abdomen
  Upper chest
- Ambulatory patients
  Abdomen
  Upper thigh
  Outer aspect of the upper arm

Special Considerations

- Cachectic patient
  Avoid the chest
  Risk of pneumothorax
- Large volumes (e.g., hypodermoclysis)
  Abdomen is usually a better option
- Large surface area
- Fluids can diffuse

Placing a SQ Line
Preparation

- Explain procedure to patient
- Prep skin with betadine and then alcohol
  23–25 gauge butterfly with adapter and Hep lock plug
- Prime tubing and butterfly with 0.5ml of saline (volume of tubing is 0.3ml)

Placing a SQ Line
Procedure

- Insert needle into SQ tissue at 45-degree angle
- Secure with opsite
- Inject medications at room temperature
- Flush with 0.5ml saline after each use
- Check site daily
- Change if inflammation or at 72 hours per policy

Subcutaneous Infusions
Methods

- Intermittent with syringe
- Infusion pump (for relatively low volume)
  Special programmable pump
  Usually uses concentrated medications (typically morphine)
- Continuous basal rate
- PCA (patient-controlled analgesia) in form of bolus
- Hypodermoclysis
  Uses typical IV infusion pump for rehydration

Subcutaneous Therapy
Appropriate Medications

- Opioids
  Morphine
  Hydomorphone
- Antiemetics
  Haloperidol
  Metochlopramide
  Promethazine

Subcutaneous Therapy
Appropriate Medications

- Sedatives/Anticonvulsants
  Lorazepam
  Midazelam
  Phenobarbital
- Corticosteroids
  Dexamethasone

Subcutaneous Therapy
Appropriate Medications

- H2 blockers
  Ranitidine
- Antihistimine
  Benadryl
  Vistaril
- Hormones
  Octreotide
- Diuretics
  Forusimide

Subcutaneous Therapy
<u>Inappropriate</u> Medications

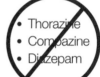

- Thorazine
- Compazine
- Diazepam

Hypodermoclysis

- Use Normal Saline or D5 1/2 NS vs. D5
- Subcutaneous tissue of the abdomen
- Infusion rate as tolerated
  May be 30 to 50cc/hour
  May be able to significantly rehydrate an individual in 24–48 hours

Subcutaneous Therapy
A Palliative Response

- In home setting

- When IV access is difficult to obtain

Subcutaneous Therapy

Selected Readings

Administration

Moriarty, D. and E. Hudson. "Hypodermclysis for Rehydration in the Community." *British Journal of Community Nursing* 6 (2001): 437–643.

Obenour, P. "Administering an S.C. Medication Continuously (Subcutaneous Infusion)." *Nursing Library,* 1998: June.

O'Doherty, C. A., E. J. Hall, L. Schofield, and G. Zeppetella. "Drugs and Syringe Drivers: A Survey of Adult Specialist Palliative Care Practice in the United Kingdom and Eire." *Palliative Medicine* 15 (2001): 149–154.

Torre, M. C. "Subcutaneous Infusion: Mon-metal Cannulae versus Metal Butterfly Needles." (Review) *British Journal of Community Nursing* 7 (2002): 365–369.

Alternative Administration Routes

Bruera, E. "Alternate Routes for Home Opioid Therapy." *Pain Clinical Updates: International Association for the Study of Pain,* 1993; 1(2).

McCaffery, M. and C. Pasero. "How to Choose the Best Route for an Opioid." *Nursing,* 2000: December.

5.6 Tube Feeding

Key Points

1. The use of feeding tubes has increased dramatically in the last decade.

   Up to 15% of patients in some nursing homes may have feeding tubes in response to Minimum Data Set (MDS).

2. Feeding tubes cause significant distress to many patients.

   Patients must be restrained to prevent them from pulling or dislodging tubes.

3. It is imperative that the physician examine the Goals of Care when considering a feeding tube.

   Feeding tubes can contribute significantly to both quality and quantity of life in some patients. Tube feeding may be indicated if it would meet the goals of addressing hunger or anxiety over declining oral intake; improving overall functional status; and bridging to a time when patient may eat again. Tube feeding is probably not indicated if it does not accomplish the Goals of Care.

4. Tube placement and complications of enteral feeding can contribute to mortality. Adverse effects of enteral feeding may outweigh any benefits.

   No published evidence suggests that tube feeding prevents aspiration; prevents consequences of malnutrition in patients with cancer, HIV/AIDS, or advanced dementia; prolongs survival of demented patients with dysphagia; prevents or promotes healing of pressure ulcers; increases resistance to infection in dementia; improves function, strength, or functional independence scores of frail elderly nursing home patients; or improves patient comfort.

5. Some families will persistently request feeding tubes despite these data. Try to support their informed decision even if it is not in concordance with medical recommendations.

6. Terminally ill patients on tube feeding may have increased need for symptom management, and their families, for emotional, spiritual, and social support.

Tube Feeding

The Palliative Response

Use of Feeding Tubes

- The use of feeding tubes has increased dramatically in the last decade
- In some nursing home units, up to 15% of patients may have a feeding tube in response to MDS
- Feeding tubes cause significant distress to many patients, who must be restrained to prevent pulling and dislodging of tubes

Role of Feeding Tubes

- Feeding tubes can contribute significantly to both quality and quantity of life for some patients
- It is imperative for the physician to examine the Goals of Care when considering tube feeding
- Tube feeding is probably not indicated if it does not accomplish the Goals of Care

Types of Feeding Tubes

- Nasogastric
  Large bore hard tube
  Silcon flexible
- Percutaneous endoscopic gastrectomy
- Open gastrectomy
- Jejunostomy

When Feeding Tubes Often Are Helpful

- Intubation and mechanical ventilation
- Mechanical obstruction in the oral pharyngeal region or esophagus
  Tumor
  Radiation and/or chemotherapy effects
- Neurological disease (such as CVA, ALS, or other degenerative disease) that affects swallowing

When Feeding Tubes Usually Are Not Helpful

- Decline in oral intake associated with progressive dementia
- Old age with declining ADL and ability to prepare food or feed self
- Nursing-home placement
- Weight loss and general debility secondary to overall declining health

Goals of Care

- Address hunger or anxiety over declining oral intake
- Improve overall functional status
- Provide bridge to time when patient may be able to eat again
- Implementation of preference stated in Advance Directive for health care

Goals of Care
Mr. Johnson

- Mr. Johnson has recently been diagnosed with an esophageal cancer and is having trouble swallowing because of the mass.

When radiation and chemotherapy induced inflammation, a PEG tube was placed as a bridge until he resumes oral intake after a few months of therapy.

Goals of Care
Mrs. Kirk

- Mrs. Kirk has experienced a severe stroke and is having trouble swallowing.

Mrs. Kirk, her family, and her doctor are following her Advance Directive for health care by placing a feeding tube for a six-week trial with the goal of relearning to swallow with speech therapy. However, she does not want permanent enteral feeding.

Goals of Care
Mr. Ascot

- Mr. Ascot has had Alzheimer's dementia for eight years.

Recently his functional status has declined: he is bed-confined, says only yes and no, is in restraints to prevent his pulling out IVs, and has declining oral intake and medications. He has "failed a swallowing test," and a PEG tube is recommended.

Consider Goals of Care

What are the Goals of Care?

- Prevent aspiration?
- Prevent consequences of malnutrition?
- Improve survival?
- Prevent of promote healing of pressure sores?
- Reduce risk of infections?
- Improve functional status?
- Improve patient comfort?

Consider Goals of Care

Prevent aspiration?

- No published evidence suggests that tube feeding prevents aspiration
- Patients still must swallow oral secretions
- The gastrostomy tube feeding with filling of the stomach can induce regurgitation and aspiration of the feeding tube contents
- No published data suggest that jejunostomy tube prevents aspiration

Consider Goals of Care

Prevent consequences of malnutrition?

- Published data have not supported the hypothesis that increased caloric intake in patients with cancer or AIDS/HIV reverses chachexia and improves survival
- Patients with advanced dementia still experience loss of lean body mass; adverse effects of enteral feedings may outweigh any benefit

Consider Goals of Care

Improve survival?

- Careful hand feeding is effective with many patients
- Dietary assistance with high caloric, easy-to-swallow foods can be helpful
- Tube placement and complications of enteral feeding can contribute to mortality
- No published data suggest that tube feeding prolongs survival in demented patients with dysphagia

Consider Goals of Care

Prevent of promote healing of pressure soresl?

- There are no published data that tube feeding prevents or promotes healing of pressure ulcers
- Bedfast, incontinent patients with feeding tubes are more likely to be restrained and probably make more urine and stool; this combination of effects may induce or worsen problems with pressure ulcers

Consider Goals of Care

Reduce risk of infections?

- It has been postulated that improved nutritional status may be associated with increased resistance to infection; there are no published data to support this in dementia
- Infection and cellulitis with the PEG tube are reported in 3–8% of all patients

Consider Goals of Care

Improve funcional status?

- Studies of frail nursing-home patients have found no improvement in function or strength with protein supplement
- Retrospective review in a nursing home found no improvement on functional independence scores of any patient during 18 months after PEG tube placement

Consider Goals of Care

Improve patient comfort?

- Patients with ALS still cough on their own secretions
- Patients are denied pleasure of food
- Patients experience discomfort from the tube and often require restraints
- Palliative-care patients rarely report hunger; when they do, small bites of food, fluid, or ice chips can usually assuage the hunger

Adverse Effects

- Aspiration   0–66.6%
- Tube occlusion   2–34.7%
- Tube leakage   13–20%
- Local infection 4.3–16%
- Approximately 2/3 of PEG tubes will need to be replaced

Conservative Management

- Stop nonessential medications
- Consider dexamethasone as appetite stimulant
- Improve dental and oral hygiene
- Position patient upright and out of bed if possible
- Assist with small, easy-to-swallow, and frequent small meals

Conservative Management

- Interventions such as these have been reported in small studies to result in a 4.5 kilogram weight gain in 50% of patients

Family Counseling

- Families experience data on tube feeding as counter-intuitive
- Some families persistently request tube feeding despite data due to cultural implication of declining oral intake

Family Counseling

After counseling about the limited benefits and the burdens of interal tube feeding, support informed decision regardless of concordance with medical recommendation.

Family Counseling

Terminally ill patients on tube feeding are eligible for hospice services; they may have increased needs for symptom management, and their families, for emotional, spiritual, and social support.

Tube Feeding

Selected Readings

Need for Physician Understanding and Leadership

Weissman, D. E. (ed). "Feeding Tubes at End of Life: The Lack of Physician Leadership." *Journal of Palliative Medicine* 3 (2000): 1–3.

Appropriate Use of Nutrition and Hydration

McCann, R. M., W. J. Hall, and A. Groth-Juncker. "Comfort Care for Terminally Ill Patients: The Appropriate Use of Nutrition and Hydration." *Journal of the American Medical Association* 272 (1994): 1263–1266.

Tube Feeding in Patients with Advanced Dementia

Finucane, T. E., C. Christmas, and K. Travis. "Tube Feeding in Patients with Advance Dementia: A Review of the Evidence." *Journal of the American Medical Association* 199; 282: 1365–1370.

Meier, D. E., J. C. Alronheim, J. Morris, S. Baskin-Lyons, and R. S. Morrison. "High Short-Term Mortality in Hospitalized Patients with Advanced Dementia: Lack of Benefit of Tube Feeding." *Archives of Internal Medicine* 161 (2002): 594–599.

5.7 Withdrawing Ventilation Support

Key Points

1. We never withdraw <u>care</u> from patients at Life's End. However, we may withdraw a <u>therapy</u> (e.g., mechanical ventilation) and increase other forms of care when the burdens of therapy outweigh its benefits.

2. Mechanical ventilation therapy is a <u>bridge of support</u> until improvement allows patient to be off ventilator. When mechanical ventilation no longer bridges to recovery, it is no longer supporting Goals of Care.

    Use available criteria to help assess whether a patient can successfully wean off ventilator support. A decision to withdraw the therapy is appropriate in an incurable or irreversible illness when it no longer advances the Goals of Care.

3. Conduct a family conference to share the prognosis, select reasonable Goals of Care, and prepare family for outcome of withdrawing ventilation.
    - Discuss patient's status in simple language
    - Explain why patient is unlikely to improve
    - Discuss options. Review any Advance Directive for guidance
    - Has patient ever discussed treatment preferences for Life's End?
    - What would patient choose if he knew he had an illness that man cannot cure?

4. Be prepared for symptoms and have a plan to control them. Have a plan for care outside of the unit if patient is stable after ventilator removed. (See "Last Hours of Life.")

5. Provide maximal support for the family during and after withdrawal.
    Offer calm, supportive presence; schedule daytime withdrawal for maximal interdisciplinary support. Meet with family after patient dies; offer to be available for questions. Consider moving patient to a private room to support family time.

6. Monitor patient frequently.
    Turn off monitors if allowable and use physical signs (e.g., respiratory rate) to guide treatment. Family and staff have tendency to stare at monitors instead of interacting and attending to patient.

Withdrawing Ventilation Support

The Palliative Response

Care versus Therapy

- We never withdraw <u>care</u> from patients at Life's End
- The burden of a particular type of <u>therapy</u> (e.g., mechanical ventilation) may outweigh the benefits
- The patient, family, and medical team may make a decision to withdraw mechanical ventilation <u>therapy</u> while increasing other forms of <u>caring</u>

Mechanical Ventilation as a Bridge

- Supports patient until he improves sufficiently to be off ventilator
- An aggressive, invasive, and potentially life-saving therapy
- Use criteria to help assess whether a patient can successfully wean off ventilator support

When Ventilation Is No Longer a Bridge

- Incurable or irreversible illnesses
- Therapy is no longer bridging to a time when patient can live without ventilator support

Clinical Considerations

Ask:
- What are the Goals of Care?
- Does ventilator support accomplish Goals of Care?

It is appropriate to withdraw ventilation therapy when Goals of Care cannot be accomplished by ventilator support.

Mechanical-Ventilator Support
Experience of Patient's Family

- One of the most stressful events in family's life
- Fatigued and overwhelmed
- Fear, guilt, and anger are common
- Usually faced with making decisions because their loved one has lost capacity
- Sometimes arguing/unable to reach consensus

Family Conference
Sharing Bad News

- Identify family members/ relationships
- Include patient if has some capacity
- Share the bad news
  Simple language
  Explain why patient is unlikely to improve
  Discuss options of care (e.g., palliative care and hospice, as appropriate)

Help Family Select Reasonable Goals of Care

- More time with family
- Transfer from ICU
- Removal of uncomfortable and nonbeneficial treatment
- Potential of conversation with patient after ventilator withdrawal, if this is a reasonable goal

Discussing Patient Preferences for Care

"Did loved one have Advance Directive?"
- Yes—Review document for guidance
- No—Do not make family feel as if you ask them to "pull the plug." Use questions such as:
  "Did patient discuss treatment preferences?"
  "What would patient choose if could speak?"
  "Would patient choose this therapy or a different kind of care if he knew he had an illness man cannot cure?"

Protocol for Withdrawal

Prepare family for outcome
- Some patients die almost immediately
- Some live a few hours to days
- A small minority has a prolonged survival

Preparation
- Determine whether family wants to be with patient during removal of support
- Be prepared for symptoms and have a plan to control them

Protocol for Withdrawal

Timing: morning is usually best
- Give family time to prepare
- Availability of pastoral and social work support

Staff support is important
- Colleagues: Important to have their support
- Nursing staff: Discuss plan and rationale

Document carefully
- Discussion
- Decisions

Protocol for Withdrawal

Alternative care plan
- Have a care plan outside ICU if patient stabilizes

Gather supplies
- Scopolamine patch overnight or several hours before withdrawal may reduce secretions
- Open face mask with moist oxygen support
- Moist wash cloth for face after removal of tube
- Suction for secretions in oropharynx after tube removed

Protocol for Withdrawal

Procedural Preparations
- IV access with flowing IV
- Draw up morphine for IV infusion
- Draw up lorazepam for IV infusion
- Turn off tube feeding 4–6 hours in advance
- Elevate head of bed
- Remove nasogastric (NG) tube and restraints
- Remove telemetry or other devises if possible

Turn off all alarms and monitors

Protocol for Withdrawal

Procedure
- Premedicate patient with morphine 2–5mg IV for dyspnea and lorazepam 1–2mg for anxiety
- Deflate cuff <u>completely</u>
- Remove endotracheal tube
- Suction mouth and oropharynx
- Wipe and clean face and neck
- Place open face mask for humidity
- Monitor and titrate morphine and lorazepam for comfort

Post-Procedural Measures

Family
- Invite to stay with patient if not already present

Comfort
- Use physical signs to guide treatment

  e.g., respiratory rate (RR) as guide for medication such as RR>16–20 morphine 2–5mg IV q1hr

- Do not use ABG, oxygen saturation or other monitoring to guide treatment

Post-Procedural Measures

Turn monitors off if policy allows
- Family and staff have tendency to stare at monitors instead of interacting and attending to patient

Consider private room
- To provide more time and privacy for patient and family

Protocol for Withdrawal

Assess
- Assess patient frequently after extubation

Support
- Be a calm and supportive presence to family
- Garner support for the family from other sources: pastoral care, social work, nursing and community
- Meet with family after patient dies
- Refer for bereavement support as needed
- Offer to be in contact with family for questions

Mechanical Ventilation

Withdrawing Ventilation Support

Selected Readings

Making the Decision

Harris, J. "Are Withholding and Withdrawing Therapy Always Morally Equivalent? A Reply to Sulmasy and Sugarman." *Journal of Medical Ethics* 20 (1994): 223–4.

Phillips, R. S., M. B. Hamel, J. M. Teno, J. Soukup, J. Lynn, R. Califf, H. Vidaillet, R. B. Davis, P. Bellamy, and L. Goldman. "Patient Race and Decisions to Withhold or Withdraw Life-Sustaining Treatments for Seriously Ill Hospitalized Adults." SUPPORT Investigators. Study to Understand Prognoses and Preferences for Outcomes and Risks of Treatments. *American Journal of Medicine* 108 (2000): 14–19.

Renauld, K. L. "Cardiovascular Surgery Patients' Respiratory Responses to Morphine before Extubation." *Pain Management Nursing* 3 (2002): 53–60.

Stroud, R. "The Withdrawal of Life Support in Adult Intensive Care: An Evaluative Review of the Literature." *Nursing in Critical Care* 7 (2002): 176–84.

Negotiating Family Conflicts

Anonymous. "Attorney for Cruzans Discusses Legal 'Odyssey'." *Iowa Medicine* 81 (1991): 249–50.

Keenan, S. P., C. Mawdsley, D. Plotkin, G. K. Webster, and F. Priestap. "Withdrawal of Life Support: How the Family Feels, and Why." *Journal of Palliative Care* 16 (2000): 40–44.

Way, J., A. L. Back, and J. R. Curtis. "Withdrawing Life Support and Resolution of Conflict with Families." *British Medical Journal* 325 (2002): 1342–1345.

Being Present When "There Is Nothing More to Do"

Walters, S. "I Took Care of It for You." *Supportive Voice*, 2002: Fall.

5.8 Death Pronouncement

Key Points

1. The time of death often dictates the provider who pronounces the death.

    Deaths often occur when primary team is unavailable (e.g., night); often the intern is the provider tasked with pronouncement. The death may be expected, with a DNAR order, or unexpected, following an unsuccessful "code."

2. Prepare for death pronouncement by reviewing nature and course of illness and immediate situation.

    Nursing staff can provide wealth of information concerning recent events, family response and dynamics, and special problems or concerns.

3. Initiate pronouncement procedures with special attention to the family relations.
    - Introduce yourself to family by your name and role ("I am Dr. ..., the doctor on call") if the family does not know you.
    - Empathize with those present ("I am sorry for your loss; this is a difficult time.")

4. Carefully follow the clinical protocol for death pronouncement.
    Document death in chart with date, time, brief statement of cause of death, and other pertinent information.
- Check ID bracelet and pulse.
    - Check pupils for position and response to light.
    - Note response to tactile stimuli in a respectful way. (No sternal rubs or nipple pinches.)
    - Look and listen for spontaneous respiration.
    - Listen for heart sound and feel for pulses.
    - Record time of death.
    - Offer to answer questions or to assist in contacting other resources.
    - Record information in chart: family present or informed; family response if indicated; notification of attending, pastoral care, social work, or others as appropriate; and name of pronouncing provider.

5. Families appreciate and respond to a respectful and kind approach to this final medical act.

    If families should contact you later, take time to ask them how family members are doing, listen carefully, and respond with empathy.

Death Pronouncement

The Palliative Response

Death Pronouncement

Circumstances of death
- May be expected with *Do Not Resuscitate* order
- May follow unsuccessful "code"

Time of death
- Can dictate provider tasked with pronouncement
- Death often occurs when primary team is unavailable *(e.g., night)*
- Often the intern is the provider available

Preparation

- Prepare to answer simple questions
- Nursing staff can provide wealth of information
  Recent events
  Family response and dynamics
  Special problems or concerns
- Assess immediate situation
  Death expected or sudden?
  Family present or notified?
  Attending notified?

Assess
Additional Requirements

- Special status
  Military category (service-connection status)
  Cause of death (e.g., Agent Orange)
- Autopsy
  Determine family request
  Consider value of autopsy
- Faith tradition
  Consider pastoral care contacts
  Honor requirements/procedures (autopsy, embalming, preparation of body)

Pronouncement Procedure
Relational Aspects

Enter
- Quiet, respectful attitude
- Ask nurse to accompany for introductions

Introduce
- "I am Dr. ..., the doctor on call"
- Determine relationships of persons present
- Inform family of purpose; invite to remain
- Offer to answer questions or to contact others

Condolences

Empathize simply
- "I am sorry for your loss…"
- "This is a difficult time"

Pronouncement Procedure
Clinical Examination

- ID bracelet and pulse
- Pupils for position and response to light
- Response to tactile stimuli
  Examine respectfully
  No sternal rubs or nipple pinches
- Spontaneous respiration
- Heart sound and pulses
- Record time of death

Follow-Up When You Are Patient's Physician

- Invite family to contact you over the next few days or months if questions arise or problems occur

Follow-Up When You Are Physician on Call

- Assure family you will report death to the attending physician, whom they may contact with questions or concerns

Death Note in Chart

- Date and time
- Name of provider pronouncing death
- Brief statement of cause of death
- Note absence of pulse, respiration, pupil response
- Note if family present or informed
- Note family response if indicated
- Note notification of attending, pastoral care, social work, or others as appropriate

Death Certificate

- Locate sample death certificate on unit
- Complete marked sections
- Write neatly in black ink
- Begin again in case of error (cross-outs often not allowed)
- Do not use abbreviations

Cause of Death
Primary and Secondary

- Cardiopulmonary arrest should <u>not</u> be the primary cause on all certificates
- Example
  Primary: *Pneumonia*
  Secondary: *Advanced*
                  Alzheimer's
                  Dementia

Cause of Death
Contributing but Not Primary

- List other illnesses possibly linked to patient's disability or service-connection (e.g., Agent Orange, Asbestosis)
- Documentation assists family to obtain benefits

Home Hospice Deaths

- Nurse pronounces death
- Certificate sent to physician to complete
- Complete death certificates promptly so that families may apply for insurance benefits and complete other paperwork

Special Considerations

Coroner's office
- Sometimes processes certificates for unexpected home deaths and ER deaths

Amended certificates
- In case of error on the certificate, appropriate clerical staff assists with processing amended certificate

Family Response

Families appreciate and respond to a respectful and kind approach to this final medical act.

Family Contacts

If families should contact you later
- Take time
- Inquire about family members
- Listen carefully
- Respond with empathy

Death Pronouncement
The Palliative Response

Death pronouncement is the final medical act.

Handle with care.

Death Pronouncement

Selected Readings

Ellison, N. M. and J. T. Ptacek. "Physician Interactions with Families and Caregivers after a Patient's Death: Current Practices and Proposed Changes." *Journal of Palliative Medicine* 5 (2002): 49–55.

Magrane, B. P., M. F. G. Gilliland, and D. King. "Certification of Death by Family Physicians." *American Family Physician,* 1997: 1433–8.

Special
Considerations

6.1 Elements and Settings of Care: Choosing a Model

Key Points

1. Most Americans die in institutions: 52% in hospitals, 24% in nursing homes, and only 24% at home. Good palliative care must occur in all settings.

2. Begin an institutional needs assessment by researching location of patient deaths in your health care system (e.g., last month, last year) and problems that occurred during the dying process.

   Examples of problems include poorly controlled symptoms, overwhelmed families and patients, lack of preparation resulting in crises and surprises, depletion of resources, and emotional and spiritual isolation.

3. Assess the strengths and resources of your health-care system for End-of-Life care.

   Assess competency, interest, and time of personnel. Assess space, administrative willingness, and financial resources of the facility.

4. Value added for patients by palliative care includes attention to suffering and to issues of meaning and purpose in the face of illness.

   Value added to staff and institutions by palliative care includes improved patient/family satisfaction, effective resource utilization, improved staff morale, increased options for disposition for patients, and improved quality of care through development of expertise throughout the institution.

5. Value added to hospices by palliative care includes increase in referrals, earlier referrals, less crisis intervention, continuity of care, and the safety net of an inpatient setting if home management is not possible.

6. Begin palliative care efforts by matching needs with available resources to choose a model: hospital consultation, inpatient unit, ambulatory clinic, nursing home, or home health care.

Elements and Settings of Care

Palliative Care

Consultation

Inpatient palliative-care units

Home hospice

Palliative Care Time Line

Therapy with curative intent

Hospice symptom Rx Supportive care

Bereavement care

Palliative Care

Presentation — 6 months — Death

Elements

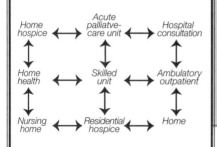

Home hospice ↔ Acute palliatve-care unit ↔ Hospital consultation

Home health ↔ Skilled unit ↔ Ambulatory outpatient

Nursing home ↔ Residential hospice ↔ Home

Continuity of Care

Last Year of Life of John, Age 83

- Home—lived alone in apartment
- Brought to ER
- Admitted to General Medical Service (progressive stage D prostate cancer)
- Transferred to palliative-care unit
- Discharged home when stabilized
  Home hospice
  Supportive care team from his church

... John's story continues

- Readmitted to palliative-care unit two months later
- Discharged to nursing home-hospice care

  Good pain control

  Friends and church members visit

  Pain worsens as progression of illness interferes with taking medication

- Readmitted to palliative-care unit

  Symptoms aggressively managed

  John dies ten days later

Settings of Care

Home	Residential	Hospital
Home Health	*Asisted living*	*Emergency ward*
Medicaid waver	*Boarding home*	*ICU*
Home hospice	*Nursing home*	*Medical wards*
	Residential hospice	*Inpatient palliative-care unit*

Deaths in USA

| **23%** | **24%** | **53%** |

Teno et. al., 1997

Assessment of Needs

- Where did people die in your health-care system last month? Last year?
- What were the problems with the care of the dying in your system?

  Poorly controlled symptoms

  Overwhelmed families and patients

  Crisis to crisis

  Lack of preparation, frequent surprises

  Resources depleted

  Emotional and spiritual isolation

Inventory of Strengths and Resources

Personnel	Facility
Physician	*Space*
Nurse	*Administrative willingness*
Social worker	*Financial resources*
Chaplain	

Competency?
Interest?
Time?

Valued Added to Patient and Families

- Suffering addressed

  Relief of suffering

  Increased capacity to bear suffering

- Issues of meaning addressed

  Assistance to find meaning and purpose in the face of illness

Value Added to Staff and Institutions

- Improved patient and family satisfaction
- Effective resource utilization
- Improved staff morale
- Increased options for disposition of patients
- Improved quality of care through development of expertise throughout the institution

Value Added for Hospice

- Increase in referrals
- Earlier referrals
- Less crisis intervention
- Continuity of care
- Safety net in an inpatient setting if home management is not possible

Choosing a Model of Care

Begin with a program that matches need with resources

- Hospital consultation
- Inpatient unit
- Ambulatory clinic
- Nursing home
- Home health

Matching Need and Resources
Palliative Nurse Consultant

- Consults in skilled unit and nursing home
- Assesses patient appropriateness for hospice
- Coordinates care of hospice patients transferred into hospital or nursing home

Matching Need and Resources
Palliative Physician Consultant

- Begins palliative medicine consult service in acute-care hospital and clinic
- Service results in improved symptom management and more referrals to hospice

Matching Need and Resources
Inpatient Palliative Unit

- Open palliative-care unit with hospital consultation to provide better palliative care to patients

Matching Need and Resources
Residential Hospice Unit

- Open residential unit to provide inpatient hospice care for patients cared for at home, in nursing homes, or in acute-care hospital

Elements and Settings of Care: Choosing a Model

Selected Readings

Hospital-Based Palliative Care

Meier, D. E. "Critical Success Factors for Hospital-Based Palliative Care Programs." Technical Assistance Series, Center to Advance Palliative Care, June 2000: 1–12. At www.capcmssm.org.

Santa-Emma, P. H., R. Roach, M. A. Gill, P. Spayde, and R. M. Taylor. "Development and Implementation of an Inpatient Acute Palliative Care Service." *Journal of Palliative Medicine* 5 (2002): 93–100.

Von Gunten, C. F. "Secondary and Tertiary Palliative Care in US Hospitals." *Journal of the American Medical Association* 287 (2002): 875–881.

Von Gunten, C. F., B. Camden, K. J. Neely, G. Franz, and J. Martinez. "Prospective Evaluation of Referrals to a Hospice/Palliative Medicine Consultation Service." *Journal of Palliative Medicine* 1 (1998): 45–153.

Linking Hospital-Based Palliative Care and Home Hospice

Bailey, F. A., J. L. Bolden, and C. G. Padgett. "There Is a Balm in Birmingham." In *Pioneer Programs in Palliative Care*, Milbank Memorial Fund, 2000.

Need to Develop Palliative Care Services in All Settings Serving the Terminal Ill

Ellershaw, J. "Clinical Pathways for Care of the Dying: An Innovation to Disseminate Clinical Excellence." *Journal of Palliative Medicine* 5 (2002): 617–621.

Goldstein, P., D. Walsh, and L. U. Horvitz. "The Cleveland Clinic Foundation Harry R. Horvitz Palliative Care Center." *Support Care Cancer* 4 (1996): 329–333.

National Hospice and Palliative Care Organization: A study about End-of-life Care. *Harris Interactive*, January 28, 2002.

6.2 Self-Care for the Palliative Provider

Key Points

1. Feelings of grief are a natural response for the medical professional in caring for patients who are at Life's End.

   It is important to develop a healthy response to stresses secondary to loss and the tragedies that can occur at Life's End.

2. "Burn-out" resulting from fatigue, multiple losses, and unresolved emotional distress can occur in the emotionally charged setting of End-of-Life care.

   The palliative-care approach assists the provider with feelings of grief and loss by offering the support of an interdisciplinary team, each of whose members brings unique strengths and abilities. The team approach recognizes unique strengths and abilities; accepts individual limits; and fosters requesting and providing assistance, thus relieving the provider from bearing loss alone.

3. Palliative care cushions the provider's sense of loss and grief by reframing treatment success.

   Palliative care reframes "failure to cure" at Life's End as success in fostering holistic healing and enabling patients to live life fully.

4. The medical provider needs to self-monitor for the depression, anger, and resentment that can result from unattended grief. Ask: "Do I still enjoy my work? Are there patients or tasks that I avoid or dread? "Do I attend to my personal health?" Self-care includes:
   - Recuperation (rest and adequate sleep)
   - Restoration (nutrition)
   - Rejuvenation (exercise)
   - Relaxation (taking all vacation time every year and regular time away)
   - Relationships (personal and professional)
   - Reflection (religion and spirituality)
   - Self-referral for concerns about physical and emotional health or substance abuse

5. Foster mentor relationships; seek mentors and be a mentor.

   Even the most skilled medical provider needs someone with whom to discuss problems, feelings, and emotions and from whom to seek guidance.

6. Self-care is an important part of being a mature and effective health-care provider. Dying persons, including dying medical professionals, do not say, "I wish I had spent more time at the office."

Self-Care for the Palliative Provider

The Palliative Response

Physician Grief Is Inevitable

Physicians care for many patients at Life's End.

Physician Grief Is Natural

Feelings of grief are the natural response to loss and the tragedies that can occur at Life's End.

Physician Grief Deserves Attention

Develop healthy responses to grief and loss.

Respect "Burn-Out"

Burn-out can occur in any field
- Fatigue
- Losses
- Unresolved emotional distress

May be more common in the emotionally charged setting of End-of-Life care

R$_X$ for Self-Care
Mutually Supportive Team

- Recognizes unique strengths and abilities; accepts individual limits
  Fosters requesting and providing assistance; relieves provider from bearing loss alone
- Understands grief as normal and expected
  Gives medical provider permission to experience feelings of grief and loss
- Provides forum to resolve inevitable conflicts

R$_X$ for Self-Care
Reframe Clinical Success at Life's End

Focus on healing versus cure.

Focus on success in healing versus failure to cure.

Clinical Success at Life's End

- Fostering holistic "healing"
- Enabling patients to live life fully
- Providing good symptom control
- Supporting patients and families

R$_X$ for Self-Care
Self-Monitor Physician Stress

Ask:
- Do I still enjoy my work?
- Are there patients or tasks that I avoid or dread?
- Do I attend to my personal health?

R$_X$ for Self-Care
R&R

Recuperation
- Make some time for adequate rest and sleep

Restoration
- Take time for meals and breaks
- Eat nutritiously
- Enjoy coffee and tea in moderation
- Stay well hydrated

R$_X$ for Self-Care
R&R

Relaxation
- Take regular time off
- Take all annual vacation time every year

Recreation
- Develop interests and creative outlets right for you at this time in your life (e.g., gardening, reading, travel, music)

R$_X$ for Self-Care
R&R

Rejuvenation
- Regular exercise is good for the body

Referral
- If concerned about your health, take time to see your own doctor

R$_X$ for Self-Care
R&R

Relationships: personal
- Take time for family and friends
- Make memories and leave legacies, daily
- Formal and informal support groups

Relationships: professional
- Seek mentors and be a mentor
- Valuable to even the most skilled medical provider
- Discuss problems/feelings; identify new solutions

R$_X$ for Self-Care
R&R

Self-**R**efer for emotional health
- If concerned about depression, discuss with your health care provider

Self-**R**efer for substance abuse
- Monitor self for abusive behaviors with substances and take action if concerned

R$_X$ for Self-Care
R&R

Reflection: religious or philosophical
- Maintain/strengthen your faith tradition
- Read or study in religion or philosophy

Reflection: personal
- Keep a personal journal
- Engage in a reflective practice (e.g., meditation, yoga)

R$_X$ for Self-Care

Develop a sense of the Transcendent.

R$_X$
Physician Heal Thyself

Self-care is an important part of being a mature and effective health-care provider.

R$_X$ for Self-Care
Remember

Dying persons—even dying physicians—seldom say,

"I wish I had spent more time at work."

Self-Care for the Palliative Provider

Selected Readings

Increasing Self-Awareness for Optimal Patient Care

Brady, D. W., G. Corbie-Smith, and W. T. Branch Jr. "What's Important to You?": The Use of Narratives to Promote Self-Reflection and to Understand the Experiences of Medical Residents." *Annals of Internal Medicine* 137 (2002): 220–223.

Meier, D. E., A. L. Back, and R. S. Morrison. "The Inner Life of Physicians and Care of the Seriously Ill." *Journal of the American Medical Association* 286 (2001): 3007–3014.

Saunders, C. "Into the Valley of the Shadow of Death: A Personal Therapeutic Journey." *British Medical Journal* 313 (1996): 1599–1601.

Scannell, K. "Writing for Our Lives: Physician Narratives and Medical Practice." *Annals of Internal Medicine* 137 (2002): 779–781.

Dealing with Grief and Loss

Baumrucker, S. J. "Palliative Care, Burnout, and the Pursuit of Happiness." *American Journal of Hospice and Palliative Care* 19 (2002): 154–156.

Keidel, G. C. "Burnout and Compassion Fatigue among Hospice Caregivers." *American Journal of Hospice and Palliative Care* 19 (2002): 200–205.

Leff, B. "Shattered All." *Annals of Internal Medicine* 132 (2000): 837–838.

Rosenblum, J. L. "Why I Still Cry. Share a Young Internist's Reflections on the Death of a Patient at the End of a Long Day." *Medical Economics Magazine* 79 (2002): 65–66.

The Palliative Response

When to Consider Palliative Care

Upon Admission:

Palliative care can often assist in improving symptom control for people with pain or other physical symptoms.

The palliative care team approach can assist you in relieving the emotional, social, and spiritual suffering patients may experience.

Palliative care can help you determine the eligibility of patients for supportive care services such as palliative care clinic, home health, and home hospice, which may provide needed assistance with home services, medications, and nurse case management.

Palliative care can help facilitate patient and family conferences to define Goals of Care, including advanced directives.

Cancer—Any patient whose cancer is metastatic or inoperable.

When to Consider Palliative Care: Side One

When to Consider Palliative Care

Heart disease
CHF symptoms at rest
EF of < 20%
New dysrhythmia
Cardiac arrest, syncope, or CVA
Frequent ER visits for symptoms

Pulmonary disease
Dyspnea at rest
Signs or symptoms of right heart failure
O2 sat on O2 of < 88%
P CO2 > 50
Unintentional weight loss

Dementia
Inability to walk
Incontinence
Fewer than six intelligible words
Albumin < 2.5 or decrease PO intake
Frequent ER visits

Liver disease
PT > 5 seconds
Albumin < 2.5
Refractory ascites
SBP
Jaundice
Malnutrition and muscle wasting

Renal disease
Not a candidate for dialysis
Creatinine clearance of < 15 ml/minute
Serum creatinine > 6.0

Failure to thrive
Frequent ER visits
Albumin < 2.5
Unintentional weight loss
Decubitus ulcers
Homebound/bed-confined

When to Consider Palliative Care: Side Two

The Palliative Response

Opioid Equianalgesic Conversion Table
(Dosing in mg unless listed)

ORAL	OPIOID AGENT	IV/IM/SQ
30	Morphine (MSC, OSR, Roxanol^{TM})	10
8	Hydromorphone (Dilaudid^{TM})	2
20	Methadone (Dolophine^{TM})	–
300	Meperidine (Demerol^{TM})	100
30	Oxycodone (Roxicodone^{TM}, OxyContin^{TM})	–
4 tabs	Oxycodone 5mg/APAP 325mg (Percocet^{TM})	–
6 tabs	Hydrocodone 5mg/APAP 500mg (Lortab5^{TM})	–
6 tabs	Codeine 30mg/APAP (Tylenol #3^{TM})	–
200+	Codeine	–

FENTANYL PATCH CONVERSION
25mcg/hour topically exchanged every 72 hours equivalent to:
Morphine 15mg IV or 45mg PO per day
Hydromorphone 3mg IV or 12mg PO per day
Percocet^{TM}/ Lortab5^{TM} /Tylenol #3^{TM} 9 tabs per day

USUAL INITIAL PCA DOSES
Morphine 1–2mg (10 mg/ml)
Hydromorphine 0.25–0.5mg (0.5 mg/ml)

- INTERVAL LOCK-OUT: Every 10–15 minutes
- FOUR HOUR LIMIT: None

1. After 24–48 hours of consistent PCA use for chronic pain, a Continuous Hourly Infusion Rate may be set at 50–75% of the daily PCA use. If a Continuous Hourly Infusion Rate is initiated, the PCA DOSE should be adjusted to 50 to 200% of this Continuous Hourly Infusion Rate every 10–15 minutes based on the patient's response.
2. Decrease the Continuous Hourly Infusion Rate as PCA use declines to avoid overmedication.
3. Never use Continuous Rate in acute pain of limited nature.

Opioid Equianalgesic Conversion Table: Side One

- Dosing tables only provide conversion estimates. Patient response may differ. Consider partial cross-tolerance when changing between narcotic agents. A well-controlled patient may require a 25% or greater dose reduction of the newly chosen agent. Opiate agonists have different durations of action, extent of oral absorption, and elimination, which may affect patient response.

- Methadone has a longer elimination half-life than duration of action and may require dose adjustment to prevent over accumulation.

- Meperidine is not indicated for prolonged therapy (greater than five days), and Normeperidine (a metabolite) may lead to seizures in patient with decreased renal function. Oral absorption of Meperidine is less reliable than other opiates and is not recommended. Its absorption, elimination, and toxicity can be affected by many drug interactions that inhibit or enhance its metabolism.

- The daily dose of acetaminophen (Tylenol) should not exceed 4 grams in a 24-hour period. This means that patients cannot use more that 8 Lortab or Tylox tablets, or 12 Percocet tablets in a 24-hour period without exceeding this limit. If pain cannot be controlled with this number of tablets, opioids not in combination with acetaminophen should be used.

- Darvon and Darvocet are ineffective analgesics and their use is discouraged.

- Constipation is secondary to opioids is common. A large bowel stimulant such as Senna or Dulcolax should be prescribed along with opioids.

- Oxycontin should not be prescribed at a less than 12-hour interval. MsContin and Oromorp should not be ordered at a less than 8-hour interval

Opioid Equianalgesic Conversion Table: Side Two

The Palliative Response

Sharing Bad News

First Step in Planning Care
- Helps develop therapeutic relationship
- Discuss agenda of patient/family first
- Let physician priorities flow naturally from the patient/family
  (e.g., discussion of resuscitation and other advance directives)

Discussion Agenda
- Physical care—Setting and level of residential care
- Social care—Family and financial issues (e.g. dependence/disability)
- Emotional care—Sources of support
- Spiritual care—Sources of meaning

Physician Role
- DO NOT DELEGATE sharing bad news
- Sharing bad news is physician's role
- Patients often accept bad news only from MD
- MD best prepared to interpret news and to offer advice

Physician Preparation
- Confirm medical facts; plan presentation
- Make only one or two main points; use simple, lay language

Setting the Stage
- Choose appropriate, private environment (Neither hallway nor
  curtain provide privacy)
- Have tissue available
- Allot enough time (20–30 minutes minimum with documentation)
- Determine who should be present
- Turn beeper to vibrate (avoids interruptions, demonstrates full
  attention)
- Shake hands with the patient first
- Introduce yourself to everyone in the room
- Always sit at eye level with patient at a distance of 50–75 cm
- Ask permission before sitting on edge of bed
- Arrange seating for everyone present if possible
  (Helps put patient at ease, prevents patient from hurrying)

Starting the Conversation
ASK: How do patient and family understand what is happening?
        What have others told them?
WAIT 15–30 seconds to give opportunity for response
LISTEN: Response may vary from "I think I am dying" to "I don't
        understand what is happening."

- How much does patient want to know?
- Ask patient if he/she wants to know prognosis
- Patient may decline conversation and designate a spokesperson

Sharing Bad News: Side One

When Family Wants to "Protect" Patient
- Honor patient's autonomy
- Meet legal obligation for consent
- Promote family alliance and support for the patient
- Ask what family is afraid will happen
- Offer to have family present when you speak to the patient (so they can hear patient's wishes about knowing status/prognosis)

Sharing Bad News
- Give a warning to allow people to prepare
- Briefly state only one or two key points
- Use simple language

STOP:
- Ask questions to assess understanding
- Recommended statement for terminal illness: "This is an illness that man cannot cure."
- Humble statement
- Leaves open the possibility of the miraculous
- Helps change the focus from "cure" to palliation and support

Do not minimize severity of news

Response to Emotions of Patient, Family, and Staff
- Be prepared for a range of emotions
- Allow time for response
- Communicate nonverbally as well as verbally (Usually acceptable to touch patient's arm)

Suggest a Brief Plan
- Medical plan (e.g., control dyspnea, home assistance to help deal with weakness)
- Ancillary support (e.g., social work visits, pastoral care visits)
- Introduce advance care planning ("Sometimes when people die, doctors try to bring them back to life... Have you considered whether you would want this or not?")
- Discuss timeline

Offer Follow-up Meeting
- When?   Usually within 24 hours
- Who?   For current and additional family members
- Why?   To repeat portions of the news
- How?   Offer to contact absent family members
          Get permission to share news if necessary
- Next meeting, upcoming decisions, suggest flexible timeline

Ending the Meeting
- ASK: "Do you have any questions?"
- WAIT
- ANSWER
- STAND—An effective way to end the conversation

Sharing Bad News: Side Two

The Palliative Response

Comfort Care in the Last Hours of Life

Admit to: Location and Initiate Comfort Care Order Set
Diagnosis: (i.e. Metastatic Lung Cancer/Pain Crisis)
Condition: Grave
Resuscitation Preferences: Do Not Attempt Resuscitation (DNAR)
                 (if not, document exact status)

Diet
- Order a diet; patient may improve and desire to taste food (select from CPRS order set)
- Full liquid instead of clear liquid (can advance if tolerated) (more palatable, easier to swallow, less likely to cause aspiration)
- May have food brought in by family
- Allow patient to sit up for meals; assist to eat

Activity
- Allow patient to sit in chair if desired and to use bedside commode
- Allow family to stay in room with patient

Vital Signs
- Minimum frequency allowed by policy
- Limit notification orders to those necessary (review options on CPRS)
- Frequent monitors can alarm patient and family
- Numbers can distract staff/family from patient

IV Considerations
- Starting is often difficult and painful, often has no benefit for patient
- Presence of edema indicates that patient is not dehydrated
- Many patients have fluid overload, edema and pulmonary congestion
- **Oral hydration is a reasonable compromise**
- **(or) If IV fluids are used, suggest a limited time trial, such as a 1000–1500 cc D5½ NS over 6 hours** (Select from CCOS on CPRS)

Subcutaneous (SQ) Line
- Small IV or butterfly needle inserted directly under the skin (often on the abdomen or thigh)
- For injecting small volumes of medicines when oral route unavailable
- Avoids burden of finding/maintaining IV access

Orders for Dyspnea
- Oxygen 2–4 liters nasal prong; avoid face mask
- Usually do not recommend monitoring oxygen saturation or telemetry
- **For persistent dyspnea, use opioids,** blow air on face with bedside fan, turn, reposition, sit up. Nebs may be helpful.

Hygiene
- Avoid Foley catheter if possible (may be helpful for hygiene in select patients, e.g., obese or immobilized patients)
- Diapers and cleansing may accomplish same thing
- Delirious patient may pull on bladder catheters
- Check all patients for impaction; suppository may be helpful
- Consider evaluation by skin-care nurse

Comfort Care in the Last Hours of Life: Side One

Notify Pastoral Care and Social Work of admission.

Avoid restraints.

Pain and Dyspnea
- Opioids are usually the most effective in this setting
- Calculate morphine equivalents used in recent past; adjust as needed
- Usually stop sustained-released medicines and use immediate-release
- Morphine concentrate 20mg/ml concentrate
  a. Start with MS 5mg to much higher dose based on recent use q2 hours. *Offer—patient may refuse*
  b. Morphine Sulfate 2–4 subq q2 hours (1/3 the oral dose) *Offer—patient may refuse*
  c. May use IV but shorter half/life and only RN can administer, difficulty with maintaining IV

Pain, Dyspnea, Anorexia, Asthenia, and Depression
- Corticosteroid can have multiple beneficial effects
- Less mineral-corticoid effect than Prednisone
- Does not have to be given in multiple doses
- Dexamethasone 4–8mg PO/SubQ breakfast and lunch

Nausea and Delirium (Phenothazines)
  a. Haloperidol 2mg PO or 1 mg SubC q2 hours, x 3 doses total or until settled, then q6–8 hours PRN
  b. Patient > 65 years of age: Haloperidol 1mg PO or 0.5 mg SubQ q2 hours, x 3 doses total or until settled
- Nausea usually requires less frequent doses

Anxiety and Seizures (Benzodiazepines)
  a. Lorazepam 1mg PO/ SubC q6–8 hours prn
  b. Patient > 65 years of age: Lorazepam 0.5 mg–1 mg PO/ SubQ q6–8 hours prn
- May be helpful with anxiety
- Exercise care as delirium can sometimes be mistaken for anxiety
- Effective against seizures only as IV or SQ and not PO

Death Rattle
- Keep back of throat dry by turning head to side
- Stop IV fluids or tube feeding
- Scopolamine patch topical behind ear q3 days
- Atropine eye drops 2–3 in mouth q4 hours or until patch effective
- Avoid deep suctioning. Family can cleanse with sponge sticks

Tips for Comfort and Safety
- Reposition, massage, quietly sit with and speak to patient
- Avoid sensory overload (e.g., TV); soft music instead
- Use bed minder in lieu of restraints to alarm if patient gets up

Assisting Family
- Advise about alerting other family members as to gravity of patient's status
- Facilitate family presence; order permission for family to visit or stay
- Arrange visits of military relatives by contacting Red Cross
- Arrange visits of incarcerated relatives by contacting Warden
- Give family the pamphlet *Gone from My Sight*

Comfort Care in the Last Hours of Life: Side Two

The Palliative Response

Guidelines for Pronouncement

Preparation before Death Pronouncement
- Be prepared to answer pertinent questions
- Nursing staff can provide wealth of information
- Know recent events, family response and dynamics, and special problems or concerns
- Assess immediate situation
  Death expected or sudden?
  Family present or notified?
  Attending notified?
- Autopsy
  Determine family request
  Consider value of autopsy
- Organ donation
  If family requests, contact organ donation counselor to discuss details
- Faith tradition
  Consider pastoral care contacts
  Honor requirements/procedures/rituals

Entering the Room
- Quiet, respectful attitude
- Ask nurse to accompany for introductions
- Introduce yourself and role: "I am the doctor on call"
- Determine relationships of persons present
- Inform family of purpose; invite to them to remain
- Empathize simply:
  "I am sorry for your loss. This is a difficult time."

Pronouncement Procedure Clinical Examination
- Check ID bracelet and pulse
- Check pupils for position and response to light
- Check response to tactile stimuli
  Examine respectfully: No sternal rubs or nipple pinches
- Check for spontaneous respiration
- Check for heart sound and pulses
- Record time of death

Guidelines for Pronouncement: Side One

Follow-Up When You Are Patient's Physician

Invite family to contact you over the next few days or months if questions arise or problems occur

Follow-Up When You Are Physician on Call

Assure family you will report death to the attending physician, whom they may contact with questions or concerns

Death Note in Chart

- Date and time
- Name of provider pronouncing death
- Brief statement of cause of death
- Note absence of pulse, respiration, pupil response
- Note if family present or informed
- Note family response if indicated
- Note notification of attending, pastoral care, social work or others as appropriate

Death Certificate

- Locate sample death certificate on unit
- Complete marked sections. Write neatly in black ink.
- Begin again if make an error (cross-outs not allowed)
- Cause of death—primary and secondary

Example: Primary: Pneumonia
Secondary: Advanced Alzheimer's Dementia

- "Contributing but not primary" section. List other illnesses possibly linked to patient's disability or service connection (e.g., Agent Orange, Asbestosis)

Documentation assists family to obtain benefits
Families appreciate and respond to a respectful and kind approach to this final medical act

If families should contact you later

Take time
Inquire about family members
Listen carefully
Respond empathically

Death pronouncement is the final medical act.
Handle with care.

Guidelines for Pronouncement: Side Two

Index

D

Darvon, Darvocet, 290
death anxiety, 194–196
death certificates, 269, 296
death pronouncement
    preparations, procedures,
        267–270
    Provider Pocket Card,
        295–296
debility, prognosis, palliative
        treatment, 99–102
Decadron, 13, 71
dehydration
    and delirium, 190
    treatments, 51–54
delirium
    described, treating, 187–191
    and insomnia, 33, 35
    during last hours of life, 97
    opioid side effect, 76
dementia
    key markers, prognosis, care
        planning, 105–109
    and tube feeding, 258
Demerol, 65, 69, 289
dentures, 46
depression
    diagnosing, treating, 199–201
    and fatigue, 18
    palliative providers', 281–282
dexamethasone
    as anti-inflammatory, 42
    as appetite stimulant, 9, 12
    for fatigue, 15, 19
    for intestinal obstruction, 59
    during last hours of life, 97
    for nausea, 40
diagnosing
    asthenia (fatigue), 17
    constipation, 22–24, 23–24
    dehydration, 53
    dyspnea, 28
    insomnia, 34–35
dialysis therapy and renal disease,
    124

diet
    for anorexia, 10
    during last hours of life, 95
    in nursing-home care,
        169–170
Difucan, 47
Dilaudid, 65, 67, 289
diuretic treatment
    for breathlessness, 131
    for edema, 133
DNAR (Do Not Attempt
        Resuscitation) orders, 91,
        95, 240, 245–246
DNR (Do Not Resuscitate) orders,
        91, 95
documentation
    advance care planning, 239,
        240
    of family conferences, 246
Dolophine, 65
dopamine antagonists, 57, 60
dosage
    opioids, general principle,
        75
    pain medications, escalation
        considerations, 69–71
dronabinol (appetite stimulant),
        13
drugs
    See also specific medication
    delirium management, 189
    prescribed in nursing home,
        170
dry mouth, 47
Dulcolax, 21, 24, 290
duragesic fentanyl patch, 67
dying process
    See also Life's End
    developing expertise in, 179
dyspnea (breathlessness)
    causes, diagnosing, treating,
        27–30
    and dehydration, 53
    during last hours of life, 96
    and pulmonary disease, 117